Supporting You and Your Combat Veteran During and After Deployment

By Doug Bey M.D.

Copyright © 2012 Doug Bey M.D.
All rights reserved.
ISBN: 1480047074
ISBN 13: 9781480047075

When a soldier comes home, he finds it hard....
....to listen to his son whine about being bored.
......to keep a straight face when people complain about potholes.
....to be tolerant of people who complain about the hassle of getting ready for work.
....to be understanding when a co-worker complains about a bad night's sleep.
......to be silent when people pray to God for a new car.
...to control his panic when his wife tells him he needs to drive slower.
...to be compassionate when a businessman expresses a fear of flying.
....to keep from laughing when anxious parents say they're afraid to send their kids off to summer camp.
....to keep from ridiculing someone who complains about hot weather.
....to control his frustration when a colleague gripes about his coffee being cold.
....to remain calm when his daughter complains about having to walk the dog.
....to be civil to people who complain about their jobs.
....to just walk away when someone says they only get two weeks of vacation a year.
....to be happy for a friend's new hot tub.
....to be forgiving when someone says how hard it is to have a new baby in the house.
....not to punch a wall when someone says we should not help others
The only thing harder than being a Soldier...
is loving one.

— George Hart

Dedicated to our warriors and those who love and support them.

Other Books by Dr. Bey

Wizard 6, A Combat Psychiatrist in Vietnam. Texas A&M University Press, 2006.

Loving an Adult Child of an Alcoholic, with Deborah Bey, RN. New York: M. Evans Publishing, 2007.

Loving a Depressed Man. New York: La Chance Publishing, 2010 *(Winner of ForeWord Review's Best Book of the Year in the Self-Help Category).)*

Acknowledgments

Thanking my family, friends, and the professionals who supported my efforts and provided input and help in creating and crafting this book is one of my greatest pleasures.

Thanks to my wife, Debbie, coauthor of *Loving an Adult Child of an Alcoholic*, who not only puts up with my writing but also encourages me to go ahead with projects (probably to get me out of her way). Thanks to my children, Cathy Ward, Barbara White, Sarah Bey, and Matt Bey, and our godson, Alvis Martin. Thanks as well to my grandchildren: Keslie and Kyle (Douglas) Ward and Audrey, Andy, and Rachel White for their encouragement. I hope my books will give you a better understanding of me and will help you remember me in years to come.

In 2006 I published a memoir, called *Wizard 6*, of serving as the First Division psychiatrist in Vietnam during 1969–1970. One positive side effect of this event was my reconnection with many of the doctors and technicians who served with me in Nam. Their input, as well as that of their spouses, provided helpful information for this book. Lt. Colonel John Hamilton, Major John Donovan, Captain Ross Guarino, Major Ed Colbach, Captain Ray Troop, Spec 4 Simon former corpsman, Spec 5 Walter "Dusty" Smith, Spec 5 Louis Stralka, Spec 4 Vincent Zecchinelli, Eric Traub, RN, who served as a combat corpsman in Vietnam, and Lt. Colonel

Bruce Capehart, who was a corpsman and career officer in the Army Medical Corps. Major John Donovan, Delta Force Vietnam, demolitions editor for *Soldier of Fortune* magazine, read the manuscript and provided his input. John and his sons, including the future soldier Sam, are all patriotic warriors who have served at the tip of the spear in combat. Command Sergeant Major Gary Huber served in Vietnam and has been active in helping veterans since his retirement from the Army Reserves.

Over my forty years of private psychiatric practice since I returned from Vietnam I've been privileged to see many veterans and their families. They provided information and, in many cases, suggestions and their own "war stories." I had Special Forces pals in Vietnam, including Major Al Breeland. I've been in contact with a number of these Special Forces heroes since Vietnam. Sergeant David Lyle, Master Sergeant Mike Jones, and Matt Donovan, all of whom served in Afghanistan, as well as a number of veterans in other specialties. Cris Ivany was a psychiatrist in Iraq who corresponded with me while serving there. Cassi Steiger Anderson and Julie Kincey were waiting wives who shared their experiences during and after their husbands' deployments. Doug Massey corresponded with me while serving as a medic/shooter with a private contracting service in Afghanistan. These individuals have shared their experiences and provided helpful input into the book.

I want to thank my literary agent, Bert Krages, for his help since I first contacted him in February 2002. He has been kind and patient with this old novice writer. This will be our fourth book together.

I also want to thank Juris Jurjevics for his friendship and for going out of his way to refer my previous manuscript to LaChance Publishing, which accepted it for publication. Juris is a Vietnam veteran, former owner of the SoHo Publishing Company, and author of *The Trudeau Vector* and *Red Flags*. The latter is a recent novel about combat in Vietnam that is based on his personal experiences as well as considerable research.

I always like to acknowledge our good friends at our "pub," Jim's Steakhouse, because we are there nearly every week and they have always supported my writing efforts. My previous three books are framed and displayed on the walls of the bar area, and there is a space waiting for this one as well. Greg, the owner, Kiley, the chief chef, Mary Jo, Chuck, Erin, Trish(es), the two Shannons, Tracy, Carmen, Stacy and Vincent, are all great people and provide a wonderful dining experience for Deb and me.

I have beaucoup medical problems and require lots of care. Thanks to Dr. Trask, my cardiologist, Dr. Hanson, internist, Dr Miller, rheumatologist, Dr. Lee, ophthalmologist, Dr. Dunkelberger, VA internist, Dr. Roszhardt, urologist, Dr. Keller, dentist, Dr. Yang, gastroenterologist, and Dr. Zander, rectal-colon surgeon (the last two can vouch that I meet the necessary qualifications to be a storyteller!).

Table of Contents

Acknowledgments v

Section I: Introduction 1

Section II: General Considerations 17

Section III: Predeployment 41
    Chapter One: Induction Changes 41
    Chapter Two: Advance Preparation for Deployment 73

IV: Deployment 89
    Chapter Three: Soldier to Warrior, Military Spouse to
    Military Waiting Spouse 89

Section IV: Deployment 111
    Chapter Four: Short—Pre-Entry--Anticipation of
    Homecoming 111

Section V: Post deployment 123
    Chapter Five: Honeymoon 123

Section VI: Normal Reactions to Abnormal
    Situations and Readjusting to Home 135

Section VII: Pathological Problems 167
    Chapter Six: PTSD, Depression, Survival Guilt, Food
    Addiction, Chemical Dependency, Sex Addiction,
    Gambling, Internet Addiction 167

VIII. Ideas for the Future 211

IX Postscript 247

X References 253

Online Resources 269

Section I: Introduction

There is concern for the mental health of our combat veterans and the welfare of their families. Thirteen soldiers commit suicide each day. As many troops committed suicide at home and abroad as were killed in combat in Afghanistan. Risk factors for suicide include: males, Caucasians, repeated tours of duty, inadequate pain treatment, failure to identify mental health problems, loss of significant relationships at home, substance abuse, inadequate treatment, fear of stigma for seeking help, fear of admitting weakness, post-traumatic stress disorder (PTSD) from combat exposure, younger age, and Reservists and National Guard. An estimated 20 percent of returning troops suffer from PTSD and only one-quarter of veterans with the condition get help. Traumatic brain injury (TBI) is reported to be under-diagnosed and inadequately treated. There is a 25 percent increase in returning veterans seeking help for substance abuse problems. The number of prescriptions for pain medicines among troops has doubled, and 14 percent of returning troops are taking an opiate pain medication of some type (95 percent Oxycontin). Twenty-eight thousand troops were discharged in a year for misconduct. Some critics allege that a good share of these soldiers suffered from mental health and substance abuse problems. There are twenty-five million veterans of the US armed forces alive today (7.5 percent are women). Veterans make up 9 percent of the total population of the United States but comprise 23 percent of the homeless population.

The majority of these unfortunate individuals suffer from mental health and substance abuse problems. Increasing cases of child abuse, divorce, chemical dependency, and mental health problems among deployed veterans and their families have been reported. Another problem with Operation Enduring Freedom (OEF) and Operation Iraqi Freedom (OIF) is the improved transportation and medical care that has resulted in more than 90 percent of wounded patients being saved. This sounds as though it should be a positive statistic, but many of the wounded in action (WIA) are grievously injured and require years of physical and psychological treatment. During World War II, two soldiers were wounded in action for every one killed in action (KIA). In Vietnam and Korea there were three WIAs for every KIA. In Iraq sixteen were sick or WIA for every KIA. Many more soldiers witnessed their buddies being killed or injured and were traumatized by seeing their horrendous explosive-induced wounds. We saw this in Vietnam. The Australian psychiatrists reported that their troops initially had a number of explosive injuries from land mines at Vung Tau. The troops' morale suffered from experiencing and witnessing these extremely debilitating wounds. Australian psychiatric casualties were lessened when the minefields were cleared and the explosive injuries were reduced.

The Veterans Administration has been criticized for not providing adequate care to returning veterans and their families. Long delays in processing veterans' compensation claims have compounded their difficulties. The number of military mental health workers has increased 60 percent since 9/11, but the troops seeking help has increased 75 percent since 2006. Soldiers have been making over one hundred thousand mental health visits/month, according to some estimates. A tenth of soldiers who've served in combat have a mental ailment, and the amount rises to one-fifth among those with a second deployment and one-third for those with three or more deployments. More than 500,000 troops have returned home in the past ten years with mental problems. In June of this year

Section I: Introduction

there were thirty-two suicides—twenty-two had been in combat and ten were deployed two or more times. By the end of 2008, 1.7 million soldiers served in OIF or OEF, and of these 4–14 percent were divorced, 12–25 percent were diagnosed with PTSD, 11–14 percent were diagnosed with TBI, and 18–35 percent had a mental health concern. The mental health services of the military are overwhelmed with the soldiers who do ask for help. There is a concern that many professionals suffer from "compassion fatigue." There is also concern that due to the great need for help and the shortage of professionals available, the military may not be screening the quality of its professional mental health caregivers adequately because of its desperation to try to meet the demand. Critics point to Major Nidal Hasan and how, seemingly, his ideology and poor performance were ignored by the military prior to his gunning down thirteen soldiers at Fort Hood.

Soldiers from the greatest generation during World War II had their reactions to combat and deployment as well, but relatively few complained or asked for help. They maintained stiff upper lips. John Wayne's macho attitude was influenced by the General George S. Patton school of psychiatry. (He recommended making fun of soldiers who claimed to suffer from battle fatigue.) For example, my wife's father was in the Bataan Death March and a prisoner of war in Japan for three and a half years. He didn't seek help from mental health counselors or the VA. That doesn't mean he didn't need help. He was an alcoholic who ended up divorcing his waiting wife. His drinking and his marital problems adversely affected his whole family.

Today's soldiers are better trained, better equipped, more motivated, probably more intelligent, and as strong as any who have ever gone to war for our country. During Vietnam men were drafted, and many lacked motivation. (On the other hand, some were highly educated prior to service. I had social work/psychology techs working for me with master's degrees, and two had PhDs). These men could have served as officers, but this would have required an extra year of duty. In recent years warriors, their families, and the general public have greater awareness of the problems that frequently develop following military training and deployment. The military is trying to change the attitude that seeking assistance implies weakness. Recent army advertisements emphasize that it takes strength for warriors to ask for help. Fourteen percent of the current military are female. Women are generally more aware of their feelings and more apt to ask for help with their problems. Their presence may help offset the old notion that equated psychological difficulty with weakness.

Having an all-volunteer army has increased the awareness of the importance of the spouse and the family. A recruit with a family is unlikely to reenlist and remain in a stressful environment for his or her spouse and kids. Family stress is one of the primary factors leading to suicide and mental health problems in deployed troops. BATTLEMIND and resiliency training programs are recent efforts on the part of the military to support troops and their families. Commanders are no longer responsible for their troops and their dependents 24/7. Spouses are not instructed what to wear or how to act. Those who have their own careers and interests and who are not devoted to furthering their partner's military career are accepted by today's military.

A major problem affecting the mental health of today's soldiers has been the experience of redeployment. Soldiers and families who've been through this process all say that redeployment is more stressful than the original deployment. Soldiers on their second tour are twice as likely to suffer acute combat stress. Seventy-five percent of soldiers on their second tour had seen someone killed or seriously injured, and 55 percent had experienced being near a hostile explosion. The all-volunteer military was instituted in 1973. The size of the total military has been reduced to one-third of

Section I: Introduction

its numbers a decade ago, and the demand for soldiers in OIF and OEF has increased. The war in Iraq has lasted longer than America was involved in World War II. Because of the reduction in force and the demand for warriors in OIF and OEF, there has been a 300 percent increase in the number of soldiers deployed to combat areas. Some men have been deployed as many as eight times to a combat zone. As one can imagine, this exerts tremendous stress on both warriors and their families. It has also become a problem in terms of recruitment and retention in the military. In fact, it is unlikely that the mental health and family problems of the military can be significantly reduced until the problem of multiple redeployments is solved. When I was in Vietnam, we couldn't imagine going back for a second tour. The majority of the troops regarded men who requested an extension or another tour as defective in some way. My cousin, who was not defective, was a career marine pilot who did two tours in Nam. He said he followed the restrictive rules of engagement (ROE) during his first tour but, on his second, he tried to kill every enemy soldier he spotted because he didn't want to come back for a third. Top military officials today have appeared confused as to an answer for the postdeployment problems of the troops and their families. Some have suggested giving troops a month leave for every three months served overseas, shortening the tour of duty to nine months, or extending the tours of duty. To further add to the confusion, other leaders suggest we may need to institute a draft in order to recruit the numbers of soldiers required and to lower the cost to the military.

One advantage veterans currently enjoy has been the universal support from the folks at home. It has been shown that this improves morale and reduces the incidence and severity of post-traumatic stress disorder among returning troops. We've learned from Vietnam that lack of support and hostility toward returning troops had an adverse effect on their health and their ability to readjust to civilian life at home. I was a major in the Army Medical Corps when

I served as the First Infantry Division psychiatrist from 1969 to 1970. I recall some antiwar psychiatrists referring to military doctors in Vietnam as Nazis who supported an unjust war through their service. The American Psychiatric Association came out with an official condemnation of the war in Vietnam. We were unjustly accused of losing the war. In 1975 our troops withdrew at least partially in response to the political pressure of the antiwar movement. The South Vietnamese were left without our support while the North Vietnamese and Vietcong continued to be supported by both Russia and China. North Vietnamese General Giap thanked Jane Fonda and the antiwar movement in the United States as well as the liberal media for their help in achieving the communist victory. Hundreds of thousands of South Vietnamese were relegated to Stalinist reeducation camps, where many died slow, painful deaths. Three million South Vietnamese boat people attempted escape, and 25 percent of them died in the effort. The Vietnam Veterans of America organization's bumper sticker slogan is "Never Again Will One Generation of Veterans Abandon Another." Like most Vietnam veterans, I am motivated to support and assist our current young soldiers. I want to do what I can to boost their morale and let them know the folks at home are behind them. I want veterans returning from deployment to receive the welcome home that we failed to receive when we came home from Nam. We know how painful it was for us to find ourselves objects of derision or being ignored by our peers and countrymen when we came back. Most of the returning Vietnam veterans kept a low profile when they got home. Veterans didn't reconnect with one another but went their separate ways. At first Vietnam veterans didn't feel welcome in the American Legion or Veterans of Foreign War posts where the World War II veterans and the Korean veterans seemed to regard us as losers. Later, President Reagan thanked us for our service and said that the soldiers who served their country should not be blamed for the mistakes of government. The country's attitude toward us changed, and we were finally recognized and honored for our service. We began to join and take part in Legion and VFW organizations. There are approximately 7.9 million Vietnam-era veterans, representing the largest percentage of the total veteran population. Currently Vietnam veterans are the senior members of many veteran groups and have assumed leadership roles in them. Desert Storm and 9/11 awakened many traumatic memories for Vietnam veterans who presented themselves to the VA with symptoms of PTSD. In 2003, 158,000 Vietnam veterans sought help for PTSD. The lack of support they received when they returned was thought to be a factor in the high incidence of PTSD among Vietnam veterans. Nam vets have been active in making sure that our OEF and OIF troops are supported, honored, and welcomed home.

In response to the obvious need for more aid for returning veterans and their families, an increasing number of military, VA, and civilian programs have been developed to offer diagnoses, treatment, and support. The BATTLEMIND and more recent resiliency-training programs are a positive step in the military's efforts to recognize and cope with the mental health needs of the troops and their families. A plethora of books have been written addressing these problems and offering information and help to veterans and their families. This is one of them. The focus of this book will be to attempt to trace the roots of the postdeployment problems that the warriors and their loved ones experience. The roots of their difficulties appear to begin during military training. The book will suggest ways these difficulties might be reduced. It is highly recommended that the new soldier and his or her loved ones read this book prior to acquiring orders for deployment.

Young troops who marry prior to or after entering the military need extra help strengthening and enriching these important relationships. Marital and family problems are a major source of stress during and following deployment. Planning and preparation are basic to the understanding and reduction of stresses associated with deployment and the postdeployment phase.

The psychological roots of the pathological problems of post-traumatic stress disorder, depression, panic disorder, suicide, chemical dependency, child and spousal abuse, divorce, and stress-related medical problems will be presented in order to facilitate recognition of these serious problems, and ways will be suggested to alleviate them with professional assistance. Readers who may have read some of my previous books know that I have been practicing psychiatry "since Christ was a corporal." Another way of saying this is that in life one progresses from tennis to golf, from golf to shuffleboard, and from shuffleboard to "the sunny room." I've made it to shuffleboard at this point. I will share some of my own "war stories" as well as those of my veteran patients and their families. In most cases these accounts are disguised to maintain confidentiality while in a few I will identify the contributor. My "voice" in writing tends to be that of a Dutch uncle with a little humor thrown in.

The information contained in this book comes from a review of the current literature, a review of online veteran assistance programs, the author's experience as a division psychiatrist in Vietnam and as a returning Vietnam veteran, interviews with a number of returning veterans from a variety of combat experiences (World War II, Korea, Vietnam, Desert Storm, Iraq, and Afghanistan) and their spouses. It includes the writer's private psychiatric practice experience working with returning veterans and their families over the years. In addition, I have a number of veteran pals with whom I correspond on a regular basis. They provided helpful insight and feedback on the manuscript as well. When case examples are provided, the individuals' identities are disguised and protected.

Reserve and National Guard troops appear to be at higher risk for mental health problems. They make up about 50 percent of the deployed troops. As a group they are probably less motivated and their deployments less anticipated. They don't live on a post and are surrounded by civilians who have little understanding of their situations. Most of their time is spent as civilians themselves. They may have to abandon their civilian jobs and suffer financial loss when their units are activated. The average age of active-duty enlisted soldiers is twenty-seven, and for officers it is thirty-five. Reserve and National Guard enlisted men average thirty-one, while officers average forty-one years of age. Ten percent of US service members are married, and about 43 percent have children. The majority of troops are from the lower and middle classes of society. Few upper-class members and the academic "intelligentsia" have served since the Vietnam era. Donna E. Shalala, secretary of health and human services under President Clinton, said of the troops in Vietnam: "The best and brightest didn't serve."

Women have served in the military and in combat for the past four thousand years. Eight hundred thousand women served in the Russian army in World War II, and 70 percent were on the front lines. As a father of three daughters, I've always been in favor of women serving in the military. I think it will help their self-confidence when they learn they are just as courageous as the male members of society. Like the women of Israel, they are unlikely to take any guff from anyone after serving shoulder to shoulder with their male comrades. Female soldiers now make up 14 percent of our military force. Over half are married. Twenty-nine thousand females are currently serving in OEF and OIF, and over 240,000 women have been deployed to these two wars since they began. We would not be able to muster a volunteer force today without the presence of women in the military. Females make the same adjustments their male counterparts do in going from civilians to soldiers with additional challenges.

There are differences between the sexes. Women have 45–50 percent less upper body strength and 25–30 percent less aerobic capacity. Female recruits have to prove themselves to what was heretofore a male organization, especially those who find themselves training and working in a traditional male role of warrior, mechanic, truck driver, construction worker, police officer, etc. Women experience more sexual harassment (11 percent prevalence) than their male comrades in arms (1.2 percent prevalence). There were 2,374 allegations of sexual harassment in 2004. In the military only 2–3 percent of cases of alleged rapists are convicted, and they only serve an average of one year in prison. One veteran Sea Bee acquaintance of mine described how her male counterparts made her carry heavy equipment, jump out of trucks, and perform other daunting physical tasks to test her as a new female member of their male "fraternity." She said she was one of a handful of women in her unit. Men who hung out with men had no problems. Women who socialized and drank with the men were considered to be loose, while those who stayed with the women were labeled "dykes." In her unit women were sexually harassed. They were expected to use profane language like the men and "cuss like a sailor." One woman went to sleep under a trailer and the men put profane signs on her and photographed her while she was sleeping. Several young women said they scored higher than most of the men on intellectual testing but still had to work harder than the males to obtain promotions. In contrast to the female Sea Bee's experience, a woman in an air force supply unit said that women in her group had it easier than the men. The men were polite and helpful to the women. "They lifted the heavier items and tried to lighten our load in general." When told about the Sea Bee's comments, she said that women who went into traditional men's assignments like construction were expected to work like their male counterparts. A female navy recruiter was told that women had to score higher to be considered for induction. Deployed female warriors have more difficulty being accepted as soldiers rather than women. If they are aggressive they are considered butch, and if they appear feminine they aren't taken seriously. Pregnancy can be a problem. Women have six weeks' leave for pregnancy in the army, and deployments are twelve–fifteen months in duration. Women seem to have more problems with guilt about leaving their children than

Section I: Introduction

men do. When women are wounded or killed it is upsetting to their male comrades, who tend to overact with aggressive behavior. Also, when women are captured their male comrades tend to forget the mission and try to save them. The VA does not recognize sexual trauma as disability. There are between seven thousand and eight thousand homeless female veterans. Postdeployment female warriors have to shift back to a nurturing feminine role. Men come home to fill their traditional roles of father and husband. Women return from what were typically masculine roles as warriors, mechanics, and truck drivers to cook, keep house and look after their children when they return home. Obviously this is a bigger adjustment.

Currently women provide some unique services for the military. They are able to search native females at checkpoints in OEF and OIF. Their nurturing qualities enable them to relate to the female population and to the children in a way that is not possible for male soldiers. They've provided observations and suggestions (giving teddy bears to children) based on their feminine nature that has been helpful in the military's effort to win the hearts and minds of the local populace. Modern antiterrorist warfare relies on developing a positive relationship with the native population. Women may have special gifts of empathy, motherly nurturing instincts, and thoughtfulness that will be an asset to our military. Women have already demonstrated that they play an important role in the military's current mission of winning a war against terrorism.

Because women are more in touch with their feelings and are better able than men to ask for help, they may find it easier in some ways to adjust to deployment. They may have more guilt about leaving their children for an extended period of time. In Vietnam women reporters seemed to cope with stress differently than men. Females relied more on sex than drugs or alcohol to reduce their stresses. Also, it seemed that they were more verbal and supportive of one another.

The military has recently changed its stance toward gays. "Don't ask, don't tell" has been supplanted by an open policy toward their service. Twenty-five countries already permit gays to serve openly in the military. The "Don't ask, don't tell policy" here in the US seemed to encourage everyone to try to act as heterosexual as possible. Because of this policy, no accurate statistics are available as to the number of gays recently serving in the military. When I was a psychiatrist with the First Infantry Division in Vietnam in 1969–1970, homosexuality was still diagnosed as an illness by the American Psychiatric Association. One day an infantryman, covered with red dust from the field, entered my psychiatric office and announced that he had been serving in combat for a year and he was gay. He denied having any psychiatric problems; he said he just wanted me to know that he was gay and he had been serving as a combat infantryman for a year. I've often thought of him over the years since then. One of my social work/psychology technicians served his first six months as a medic with 2/28 the infantry battalion in the field. I didn't learn until years after Nam that he was gay. He said that being gay was a nonissue in a combat unit, although he did meet some gays in Nam. He reported that he was able to keep busy with school and work after he returned home, but he felt isolated because people were down on Vietnam veterans, and being gay and not out of the closet compounded his feelings of estrangement. Some OIF veterans who are gay said that they felt estranged by the "Don't ask, don't tell" policy. They agreed that they couldn't really be themselves unless they were out of the closet and open about their homosexuality. Military policy at the time prevented them from doing this.

From my experience, nearly all returning veterans (male, female, gay, and straight) and their families are likely to have adjustment problems when they come home. Men have difficulty recognizing their feelings and being able to talk about them. If you ask most men how they are feeling, they will tell you what they are thinking.

Section I: Introduction

Women are by far the biggest consumers of health care in civilian life because men are reluctant to seek help. Men tend to try to solve their own problems through compulsive behaviors. Female soldiers may serve as role models in the military for expressing feelings and being able to turn to professionals for assistance.

This book is written for the female as well as the deployed male soldier and the waiting male spouse with children as well as the waiting wife. Parents of deployed military children may gain some insights into their experiences and adjustments from reading this book. However, since the majority of deployed soldiers are male and the bulk of waiting spouses are female, as a rule, I will tend to refer to the overseas soldiers in masculine terms and the waiting spouses as female.

Every soldier in the military today, regardless of branch or if they are a reservist or a member of the National Guard, should prepare for the likelihood of deployment. Their dependents at home should anticipate their loved ones departure for combat duty as well.

A positive attitude toward deployment will help reduce some of the stresses that accompany this period for both the soldier and his family. This book is written to help warriors and loved ones gird their loins for hardship duty and the adjustments they will necessarily be required to make before, during, and after deployment. This book is written with the hope that men or women entering the military and their loved ones will read it to prepare themselves for their future experiences. It is aimed at helping them anticipate and reduce the stresses they are likely to experience. Reading this information in advance will not completely alleviate the stresses that the new recruit and his family will face adjusting to the service deployment and postdeployment, but it may lessen some of the problems. For example, if your doctor gives you a pill and tells you that it may cause dry mouth, constipation, hot flashes, and blurred vision, this information will not prevent you from getting dry mouth, constipation, hot flashes, and blurred vision. Nevertheless, the foreknowledge of these symptoms lessens the anxiety experienced when any of these side effects develop. In the same way, discussing the likely reactions to receiving orders for deployment, deployment, and then postdeployment will not prevent those experiences, but knowing about them in advance may reduce the stresses associated with them and help you and your loved ones in your efforts to cope with these changes.

This book is not a substitute for professional help. It is impossible to address all of the potential adjustment problems individuals may run into as they enter the service, go through deployment and a combat/separation-from-home experience, and then readjust to home and family. There are wide differences in childhood experiences that influence their adjustments. Ethnicity, sex, age, branch of service, military occupational training, who trained them, their spouses' backgrounds, the support they and their spouses receive, whether they are retiring from the military or remaining in, whether they lost close friends, and whether they sustained injuries during deployment are also factors. There are a myriad of variables that we are unable to include in this book. I personally believe that professional coaching is good for all of us and particularly individuals who are making adjustments in their lives. Old-timers may say that most veterans return from service and go on with their lives without help, but this doesn't mean the adjustments they made were the best and that they couldn't have done better with a little assistance. This book does discuss the difficulty men, particularly those in macho professions (military, police work, firemen, etc.), have asking for help and how their resistance to seeking professional advice can be lessened.

Suicide rates, divorce, child abuse, PTSD, chemical dependency, homelessness, and addiction to the Internet are all increasing despite more government funding, media attention, and professional manpower expended toward trying to help veterans and their families. A shortage of professional caregivers, especially those who are experienced in working with members of the military and their families, continues to exist. There is also a resistance on the part of warriors and their dependents to seek professional help. Some of this is due to the stoicism and feeling that one should take care of one's own problems that are part of being a warrior. Part is due to the feeling that mental health issues could harm security clearances or put the soldier's military advancement at risk. In addition, the treatments for PTSD, chemical dependency, Internet addiction, depression, marital dysfunction, child abuse, etc., have not been quick or universally effective. It appears that no one has the answer as to how we can prevent the adjustment problems of veterans and their families at this point. There are multiple treatment approaches suggested and being applied for the treatment of PTSD. There is currently no gold standard, which suggests that we don't know how to best treat this common disorder.

The author offers some ideas as to how treatment results might be improved. The military has perfected the rapid conversion of civilians into warrior-killers. The defenses of stoicism, suppression of feelings, suspension of guilt, and hypervigilance persist in civilian life during the postdeployment period. Why couldn't the same organization develop programs to convert warriors back into civilians? Another important change would be for top military leaders to encourage men to be more open about their problems, to urge commanders to identify problems earlier, and to pay more attention to the difficulties experienced by veterans and their dependents during postdeployment. The writer suggests a somewhat radical approach of tracing back the roots of the commonly observed problems among veterans and attempting to nip them in the bud during the predeployment training period. Mental health professionals in the combat areas may be more effective if they utilized modern technology to monitor the stress levels of the units and to then consult with those who were experiencing stress (and learn from those who were coping well). It would be helpful to have senior mental health professionals whose rank would permit them to consult and influence the higher-ranking field officers regarding the mental health issues of the troops. The author suggests mental health providers in the combat area might, in addition to helping with the immediate problems, also focus on possible postdeployment problems of their clients. Finally, the book discusses the difficulties the VA has in evaluating the psychological problems of returning veterans. Without an object measure like a blood test or x-ray, examiners must rely on the army medical records, the history the patient gives, the symptoms described by the veteran and his family, and the examiner's appraisal of the warrior when he interviews him. The author suggests that veterans who have served in the same unit and at about the same time might be the best judges of the soldier's actual combat history. Theses men could be paid to review the soldier's claims and make a final judgment as to their validity. Other veterans are likely to be empathetic and lean in favor of helping the warrior but would also be able to pick up wannabes and malingerers who feign battlefield experience.

Section II: General Considerations

With the possible exclusion of the upper class and the "intelligentsia," who have stayed aloof from serving since Vietnam, the military represents a cross section of America. My definition of "intelligentsia," by the way, is individuals who are educated beyond their intelligence. As I write I am picturing a young female reader whose husband has joined a reserve unit or the National Guard or enlisted in one of the branches of the military. As noted in the introduction, 14 percent of the troops are female, and there are male spouses whose wives are serving overseas. There are military couples who are both serving. The Servicemembers Legal Defense Network (SLDN) reports sixty-five thousand gays are serving in the military. Finally, there are parents who are concerned for their children who are in uniform. Hopefully, the reader will overlook my tendency to address the reader as a civilian female and understand that those who don't fit this stereotype will also benefit from the information and advice contained in this book.

Childhood and Background of the Individual Soldier

When I think of the individual soldier these days, a multitude of images come to mind. A range of ethnic, economic, psychological, sexual, intellectual, spiritual, and varied backgrounds exist among enlisted and officer personnel. Some are regular military while others are reservists or National Guard members. An eighteen-year-old, male, single, ethnic minority person from a large urban area who enlists is in quite a different place from a thirty-three-year-old, female, college graduate reservist who is married and grew up in a rural environment. Veterans since 1973 are professional soldiers who have chosen to serve. They are different from the drafted troops during the Vietnam era. I assumed that highly motivated, well-trained Special Forces troops would be anxious to be deployed as opposed to, for example, a reservist who may have signed up for the money and the educational benefits. I've learned from my conversations with Special Forces NCOs that this isn't always the case and that it is impossible to know how any individual will react to danger until he is actually exposed to it. Even seemingly well-trained, elite troops may try to evade or even quit the military to avoid deployment in some instances.

Obviously the information in this book will not apply to every reader at all times. I've tried to keep the wide range of backgrounds, ethnicities, sexes, rank, marital statuses, and educational backgrounds in mind, but it is impossible to provide specific counsel appropriate for every reader in all instances. Just take what is useful to you and skip information that doesn't apply to you or your family.

I will follow the KISS (keep it simple stupid) principle with my writing rather than try to be academic (the "intelligentsia" won't be reading this anyway). Karl Menninger was my teacher and role model during my psychiatric training. He hated jargon. He said if we couldn't convey what we had to say in words that were understandable to a Kansas farmer then we didn't know what we were talking about. For example, Dr. Karl had one of the residents assume the role of a ward physician with a teenage patient who acted up and was put in seclusion on the ward. Dr. Karl played the part of this Kansas farmer father. "How's my boy, Doc?" Dr. Karl asked. "He's making progress," answered the resident playing the role of the ward doctor. "Progress?" queried Dr. Karl. "What's that—some kind of beads?" During my forty-plus years of practice, I've sent each of my new patients a letter in lay terms containing the gist of our initial consultation. I've tried to follow Dr. Karl's recommendations writing to my patients and continued the same tack in this book.

Considering Marriage

Failed marriages are common in civilian life and are even more prevalent in the military. Over 60 percent of marriages in which one member is deployed end in divorce. Because of this statistic, I feel it necessary to include a section focused on marital choice and enrichment. It is important to make your relationship a top priority in your life. To coin a saying from Alcoholics Anonymous, "Make it first to make it last."

Let's assume that you are considering marriage or have recently tied the knot. I would hope that you have thought seriously about the commitment you are contemplating or have just made and that you have chosen your mate at a time in your life when you are self-supporting and happy living independently on your own. Marrying someone because you are lonely or need another person are motives that lead to difficulty.

It would be helpful to seek the counsel of your religious leader or a professional marriage counselor to discuss what a good marriage entails. Find a seasoned military couple who have a happy marriage and ask them if they would mentor you in your relationship. If your parents have a good marriage, they could provide role models and counseling. If you are going to ask for advice then listen to what the adviser says and be willing to accept information that may go against your own urges and wishes. For example, you may have made the decision to marry immediately and then hear from your mentor why you should wait. That's why you are turning to an experienced person. Don't ask for advice if you are really asking for the person's blessing for your decision or someone to share the responsibility for your decision.

Military marriages are more likely to fail than civilian marriages because of a number of factors. Most recruits are single when they join but marry before the end of their enlistment and most have children earlier than their civilian peers. This means that a large number of young individuals, poorly prepared for marriage and parenthood, impulsively tie the knot and then face severe stresses military life brings to their relationships. Military couples experience frequent geographical moves, lengthy separations, dangerous and stressful assignments, and financial pressures. An army private first class's pay and benefits comes out to approximately $1,450.00/month. (A household with two occupants is eligible for food stamps if the income is less than $1,579.00.) Military housing is frequently old, and in the case of regular army troops, occupants live on crowded posts surrounded by other young couples who are ill prepared for marriage and parenthood. The military has a reputation for infidelity. At Fort Knox the enlisted housing was referred to as Peyton Place because of the rampant infidelity occurring there. A flight surgeon in Florida told me that the Strategic Air Command (SAC) pilots would buzz their own houses when they returned from a mission to alert anyone who was there having an affair with their wives. Sergeants told me horror stories of men coming home to wives who were unfaithful, pregnant, and who had spent all of the warrior's savings while they were deployed. The NCOs described examples of spousal abuse and even murders committed by returning troops.

Young couples are frequently motivated by sexual urges. They may not really know the person they think they love and instead project an idealized version of themselves onto them and then love that projected image. They may act impulsively without realizing how damaging infidelity is to a relationship and to the trust that is basic to a good marriage. This is why it is so important to get an outside, objective opinion of the relationship and the advice of mature couples who are happy in their marriages. Good mentors will help you and your spouse realize how much effort is required to keep a relationship viable.

Make a self-assessment of your readiness to marry. Are you able to live independently and be happy on your own? Is the person you are attracted to independent and happy on his or her own? Do you share common interests, ideals, religious beliefs, and goals in life? Are you good friends? If both parties begin to contemplate marriage, they would likely benefit from educational materials and instruction about a committed relationship—instruction as to how couples strengthen their bonds, how to communicate in a relationship, how to disagree, the importance of common interests, making decisions together, financial planning, budgeting together, building and maintaining trust, sexual relations in marriage, and parenting. These are things you can learn from reading books on marriage, premarital counseling from a professional or a religious leader, mentoring by a happily married couple, and by discussing them with one another. A huge help for solving problems in a marriage is the ability to analyze conflicts psychologically.

Can you think psychologically and discuss situations in depth? We all have patterns of coping we develop during childhood to cope with stresses we encounter. These are carried over into our adult life. Usually they do not cause major problems, but they influence our actions and may cause us to overreact to what may seem trivial situations. These emotional reactions are confusing to our partners. If we can reflect and discuss them, we can figure them out and prevent conflicts in our relationships. For example, a young man grew up in a family where his mother frequently accused his dad of infidelity. He disliked his father and thought he was a selfish, mean individual. When he reached adolescence, he started following his dad and trying to catch him in the act. Instead he discovered that his father was not unfaithful, his mother was paranoid, and her accusations were products of her delusional thinking. Then he was angry with his father for putting up with his mother's false statements. This young man got a job in a bank and ended up marrying an attractive young woman who worked there as a teller. On their honeymoon the fellow decided to take a wastebasket from their motel room to the Dumpster outside. His new bride asked, "Where are you going, honey?" He blew up and shouted, "It's none of your damn business where I'm going. I'll do what I want to do and it is none of your concern!" The young woman wondered what sort of crazy person she had married. They came to me seeking help with their relationship. We sorted out the roots of the groom's emotional outburst, and they were both able to understand why he reacted as he did. I told the bride she didn't need to walk on eggshells, it was his problem, but there were topics that were emotional land mines for him and she could expect an overreaction if they came up from time to time. The important thing was that they were able to reflect on the source of the upset and discuss it with each other. I told the bride that she probably had patterns from her own childhood and there were likely topics that she was sensitized to as well. Like this couple, you may need to seek professional assistance to figure out the hot spots in your relationship initially. But, if you put your minds to it, you will be able to identify your own childhood patterns and see how they affect your adult relationships. It isn't that complicated, and it can be fun. It leads to a deeper and more interesting relationship in the long run.

Virginia Satir, the famous family therapist, suggested that couples begin their discussions with the statement "I feel," because only you know what you feel and so you are always right in what you are going to say. Also, by starting out your statement in this manner, you are not accusing your partner and will not put him or her on the defensive. For example, when you say, "When you come home and immediately go get a beer and sit in front of the television, I feel as though I am not very important to you and it makes me sad." This is better than saying, "You selfish SOB, how about giving me some attention?" The latter statement is likely to evoke a defensive response, such as, "Give me a break. I've been breaking my butt all day to earn a paycheck. I just want some peace and quiet and to get away from your griping." By the way, dinnertime is the peak time for marital conflict. Both parties are tired and want the other to nurture and feed them at the end of the day. The wife is looking forward to the husband's coming home and relieving her of some of the demands from the children and helping out around the house. The man is drained from his work and looking forward to being coddled and fed by his wife. As a result, both end up being frustrated and angry with the other for not meeting his or her dependency needs. When this is the case, we suggest they recognize what is going on and find some activities to occupy the children while they sit down and have a snack and discuss the events of the day together.

Marital and family problems are a major factor in the development of mental health problems among deployed troops. On the other hand, a good marriage and loving support from home help warriors cope with the adversities of a hardship tour.

Special Stresses for Special Groups

Women in the Military

Of the approximately twenty-five million veterans of the US armed forces today, 7.5 percent are women. Women have served in the military and in combat for the past four thousand years. Dr. Mary Walker received the Medal of Honor as a physician in the Civil

War. During the War Between the States, four hundred women cross-dressed as men in order to serve. In World War I, thirty-six thousand women served as nurses, translators, and secretaries, and two hundred lost their lives. These women were not given military rank and were not recognized as veterans. Eight hundred thousand women served in the Russian army in WWII, and 70 percent were on the front lines. Over four hundred thousand served in the United States during WWII and were granted limited rank and after the war achieved some permanent, but limited, status. As a father of three daughters, I've always been in favor of women serving in the military. I'm certain deployment would boost their self-confidence when they learn they are just as courageous men. Like the women of the twenty-five other countries that have women serving in combat, they are unlikely to take any guff off of anyone after serving in shoulder to shoulder with their male comrades under fire. Female soldiers now make up 14 percent of our military force. The air force has the highest percentage (20 percent) and the marines the lowest (6 percent). The army and navy each have 14–15 percent. Over half are married, twenty-nine thousand currently serve in OEF and OIF, and over 240,000 have been deployed to these two wars since they began. We would not be able to muster a volunteer force today without the presence of women in the military. Females make the same adjustments their male counterparts do in going from civilians to soldiers—and they face additional challenges.

As noted previously, women have 45–50 percent less upper-body strength and 25–30 percent less aerobic capacity. However, most of us have seen strong, athletic women who are superior physically to weak, out-of-shape men. CSM Huber points out that there are different physical standards by age in the military, so why not for the sexes? Women were initially excluded from the artillery because they couldn't lift the 105mm howitzer shells, but CSM Huber notes that two men load the shells and a third tamps it into the barrel on a gun crew, and two women could easily lift a shell.

Female recruits have to prove themselves to what was heretofore a male organization, especially those who find themselves training and working in a traditional male role of warrior, mechanic, truck driver, construction worker, police officer, etc. It reminds me of women in sports. When I was in high school there were few sports for women. Now women compete successfully in all sports, including, in some instances, football, boxing, and wrestling. The records for women in the Olympics keep improving. Expectation plays a large role in what women are capable of doing. Sergeant Sherri Gallagher won the army's Best Warrior Soldier this year competing in hand-to-hand combat, urban orienteering, detainee operations, casualty evaluation, weapons familiarization, and night firing.

Military service is generally more stressful for women than for men. Women experience more sexual harassment (11 percent prevalence) than their male comrades in arms (1.2 percent prevalence). There were 2,374 allegations of sexual harassment in 2004. In the military only, 2–3 percent of alleged rapists are convicted, and they serve only one year on average. Sexual trauma predisposes individuals to PTSD.

One veteran Sea Bee described how her male counterparts made her carry heavy equipment, jump out of trucks, and perform other daunting physical tasks to test her as a new female member of their male "fraternity." She said she was one of a handful of women in her unit. Men who hung out with men had no problems. Women who socialized and drank with the men were considered to be loose, while those who stayed with the women were labeled "dykes." The See Bee confirmed that, in her unit, women were sexually harassed. They were expected to use profane language like the men and "cuss like a sailor." One female soldier went to sleep under a trailer and the men put profane signs on her and photographed her while she was sleeping. Several young women said they scored higher than most of the men on intellectual testing but still had to work harder than the males to obtain promotions.

A female navy recruiter was told that women had to score higher to be considered for induction.

Women are less likely to have problems from chemical dependency or legal difficulties (for fighting, etc.) than their male counterparts. Some deployed female warriors said they had more difficulty being accepted as soldiers rather than women. If they are aggressive they are considered butch, and if they appear feminine they aren't taken seriously. Civilian women threaten suicide more frequently than men but kill themselves less often. Twice as many women commit suicide when deployed to OIF or OEF than back in the United States. Women veterans are three times more likely to commit suicide than their civilian counterparts.

Pregnancy can be a problem. Women have six weeks leave for pregnancy in the army and deployments are twelve-fifteen months in duration. Pregnant combat veterans are twice as likely to have PTSD as nonpregnant soldiers. Women seem to have more problems with guilt about leaving their children than men do. Servicewomen have a higher early discharge rate than their male comrades.

This is the first time in history where a significant number of females serving in the US military have been wounded or killed. This is a new experience for our civilian population. Female deaths and injuries are particularly upsetting to their male comrades, who tend to overact with aggressive behavior. Also, when women are captured, their male comrades tend to forget the mission and try to save them.

There are between seven thousand and eight thousand homeless female veterans. Postdeployment female warriors have to shift back to a nurturing feminine role. Men come home to fill their traditional roles of father and husband. Women return from what were typically masculine roles as warriors, mechanics, and truck drivers to cook, keep house, and look after their children when they return home. Obviously this is a bigger adjustment.

Currently women provide some unique services for the military. Turret gunners are usually women because they've shown higher aptitude for this position. Female soldiers are able to search native females at checkpoints in OEF and OIF. Their nurturing qualities enable them to relate to the female population and to the children in a way that is not possible for male soldiers. They've provided observations and suggestions (giving teddy bears to children in Iraq) based on their feminine nature that has been helpful in the military's effort to win the hearts and minds of the local populace. Modern antiterrorist warfare relies on developing a positive relationship with the native population. Women may have special gifts of empathy, motherly nurturing instincts, and thoughtfulness that will be an asset to our military. Women have already demonstrated that they play an important role in the military's current mission of winning a war against terrorism.

In Vietnam female reporters seemed to cope with stress in the combat area differently than men. They relied more on sex than drugs or alcohol to reduce their tension. At the same time, they were more verbal and supportive of one another.

The same delays, professional staff shortages, and difficulties obtaining treatment apply to both female and male veterans, but there are fewer professional services and facilities available for women in the VA system. New ones are being built, but currently treatment services for female veterans are scarcer than for the men. The VA does not recognize sexual trauma disability compensation.

Race

Our military has been integrated since the Korean War. It is representative of the melting pot culture of the United States. In Vietnam the number of black officers did not reflect the number of blacks in service. In recent years the military has become an equal opportunity employer. Veterans reflect this diversity:

White—80.0 percent
Black—20.9 percent
Hispanic—5.6 percent
Asian/Pacific Islander—1.4 percent
American Indian/Alaska Natives—0.8 percent
Other—1.3 percent

Gays in the Military

Twenty-two of twenty-five NATO countries permit gays and lesbians to serve openly in the military. Britain, France, and Russia do, for example. Until recently the United States has had the "Don't ask, don't tell policy" that seems to encourage everyone to act as heterosexual as possible. Because of this policy, no accurate statistics are available as to the number of gays currently serving in the military (except for the SLDN report of sixth-five thousand currently serving). Just recently the United States has joined the majority of NATO forces by permitting open service for gays and lesbians. When I was a psychiatrist with the First Infantry Division in Vietnam during 1969–1970, homosexuality was still diagnosed as an illness by the American Psychiatric Association. One day an infantryman, covered with red dust from the field, entered my psychiatric office and announced that he had been serving in combat for a year and he was gay. He denied having any psychiatric problems. He said he just wanted me to know that he was gay and he had been serving as a combat infantryman for a year. I've often thought of him over the years since then. One of my social work/psychology technicians served his first six months as a medic with 2/28 the infantry battalion in the field. I didn't learn until years after Nam that he was gay. He said that being gay was a nonissue in a combat unit, although he did meet some gays in Nam. The other technicians suspected that he was gay but weren't bothered by his orientation. The medic reported that he was able to keep busy with school and work after he returned home but he felt isolated because people were down on Vietnam veterans, and being gay and not out of the closet compounded his feelings of estrangement. I asked some gay veterans to give me their input regarding their experiences in the military and in combat for inclusion in this book. Gay OIF veterans said that they felt estranged by the "Don't ask, don't tell" policy. They agreed that they couldn't really be themselves unless they were out of the closet and open about their homosexuality. Recent changes have permitted open enlistment and retention of gays in the future.

Faith

This is not an effort on my part to impose my religious views on the reader. However, there is objective evidence that a strong religious faith can be a great source of strength for young married couples, soldiers in the field, and to parents who are trying to provide guidance for their children. The statement that couples who pray together stay together contains wisdom. Religion provides thousands of years of practical guidelines for living. Young couples can benefit from the structure provided by their belief system as well as the fellowship, role modeling, and counsel of couples who have good relationships and who have weathered stresses to their marriages over the years. It has been shown that individuals who have a strong faith are able to cope with stress better than those who do not. In my conversations with combat veterans, the idea that there are few atheists in foxholes probably is true. Men faced with their own mortality tend to turn to faith in a higher power. (It isn't always true, however. My father-in-law said he could hear the soldiers in the next foxhole on Bataan praying out loud just before they took a direct artillery hit and were killed. This event caused him to stop praying.) Soldiers with a strong faith did better withstanding Chinese brainwashing in Korea, and prisoners of war in Vietnam who had a committed belief system did better as well.

In addition to providing strength to face adversity, a religious commitment provides fellowship and support from other individuals who are trying to improve themselves. It helps young parents by providing instruction and moral guidance for their children. It gives them fellowship support by including them as part of the church family. Getting involved in a religion and choosing a faith is an individual choice, but it's one I believe should be seriously considered by young couples who are contemplating marriage.

Some General Principles of a Committed Marriage

The choice of a marriage partner is one of the most important decisions of anyone's life. It is a lifetime commitment. It makes the difference between a happy, fulfilled, secure life and one that is miserable and stressful. It should not be entered into lightly and certainly not on the basis of hormones, loneliness, or wanting a substitute parent. It is important for young troops to avoid making any impulsive decision prompted by enlistment or deployment.

I'm not holding myself up as an ideal example in this regard. I married at a young age for irrational reasons (she had a high IQ, which was valued by my parents), and we didn't particularly care for one another at the time we tied the knot. I was a type A, compulsive workaholic, and I made the poor rationalization that a bad marriage would permit me to put more time and energy into my work. My ex wasn't happy with me throughout the marriage and periodically told me to leave. Eventually, when the children left home it was apparent that we had no relationship, and when she once more told me to leave, I did. One of my psychology/social work techs in Vietnam told me that he married just before coming to Nam and many years later his first wife left him, telling him that she stayed because she felt sorry for him for being in Vietnam. He is now happily remarried. A good many of my comrades in Vietnam are divorced and now remarried. I'm in the same boat. I was more mature and put more thought into the choice of my second wife. We've had a very happy marriage for over twenty years. Deborah is my office nurse and coauthored the book *Loving an Adult Child of an Alcoholic* with me in 2007. The recommendations below are based on my current relationship, which is a good one.

One of my psychiatrist friends who served with me in Vietnam said this section of the book came off as a little "preachy." I agree. It is what I call my "Dutch uncle" approach. I'm trying to help you young couples think about your choice of marital partners and once you make a commitment to do all you can to keep it going. This is not a self-help guide for marital enrichment, but books of this type are available. I would strongly urge young couples contemplating marriage to read books about marriage, consult with your religious leaders, seek professional guidance, and find a happily married couple in the service to serve as a mentor to help you with your decision making and your marriage if you decide to make that commitment. Here are a few general principles that I believe will help strengthen a marriage.

- Don't take your partner or the relationship for granted. Marriage is a sacred bond and a lifelong commitment to one another. Keep this in the forefront of your minds. Because of the importance of your relationship to one another, you should never say anything that knowingly hurts or upsets your partner and, if you inadvertently do, apologize immediately.

- In adolescent love we project our ideal image onto the other person and love ourselves in them. We fantasize that this is an ideal person who will meet all of our needs. They will rescue us from our unhappy life situation and we will have a problem-free relationship. This type of "puppy love" is not reality and ends in disappointment and frustration.

Utilize the help of outside observers to evaluate your partner more objectively.

- If there were previous relationships, forget them. The only thing that counts is that you love each other now. Remember no one can *make* someone love him or her. Love must be given.

- Don't confuse your present relationship with bad ones from the past. In other words, don't get mad at your partner because he or she reminds you of a past bad experience.

- Commitment and trust are important components of a successful marriage. Jealousy can destroy a relationship.

- Knowing that your partner loves you and that what he or she says is a product of that love, you can accept suggestions from him or her as being in your best interest. For example, if a spouse suggests a diet, you accept the advice because you know it is said out of concern for your health and well-being. If you can do this, you will be stronger as a couple than you would be as two individuals. You can help each other overcome shortcomings in yourselves without becoming defensive.

- Having a person who knows everything about you and still loves you is a situation that is good for your self-esteem and mental health. This is one of the cures for "toxic shame" described by John Bradshaw in his books for adult children of alcoholics.

- Pay attention to the little things that irritate your partner and correct them if possible. For example, if your wife doesn't like to see the lid up on the toilet, make an effort to put it down. If one of you is upset by the other's messiness, learn to be neater. These are little things, but they add up in time and lead to bigger irritations. Also, by paying attention to your partner's wishes, you are showing your respect and love.

- Do little things daily to show your love. Small kindnesses add up. Leave a loving note in the bathroom, under a pillow, or in a briefcase. Do little things you know will please your spouse.

- In the 1940s there was a song that said to "Accentuate the positive, eliminate the negative, and don't mess with Mr. In between." This is good advice for your relationship.

- Encourage your spouse to grow and to be all he or she can be. You are a team. Avoid the tendency in the military to be authoritarian and to try to control or boss your spouse around.

- Don't try to change your spouse. The only person you can change is yourself. When problems arise, determine what you are doing that is contributing to the problems and correct your behavior.

- Focus your attention and affection on your spouse. Commitment to the relationship is paramount. Neither of you should doubt or worry about the other's fidelity while you are separated during deployment. The military is famous for rumors, and both parties will be exposed to stories of infidelity overseas and at home. Ignore what you hear through the grapevine and have faith in your partner's fidelity.

- Discuss decisions regarding finances, home management, the children, and day-to-day problems together and arrive at mutually agreeable solutions.

- When voicing your unhappiness about something, use "I" statements in order to avoid accusing or putting your spouse on the defensive. For example, "When you come home, get a beer, and then sit down in front of the television without speaking to me or the children, I feel ignored and unimportant. It makes me feel sad." Only you know how you feel, and so you are always right about your feelings. This is not accusing your partner and should not elicit a defensive response. You are merely reporting how his actions make you feel.

- Try to figure out what makes you each tick psychologically. Discuss your childhood experiences and how the patterns of behavior you developed as a child to cope carry over into adult life and influence your current actions. This may seem foreign to the male spouse, but it is a learned talent that will pay off in solving your problems and in developing a deeper and more interesting relationship. For example, "My dad was an alcoholic when I was growing up, and we could never count on him to make it to ball games or school activities. We walked around on eggshells, never knowing what he was going to do. Because of this I have a hard time trusting or depending on others, and I tend to be anxious when things are going well, because I anticipate that a crisis is going to occur." He may respond, "Oh, now I see why you are tense when there seems to be no reason to be anxious, and I see why you anticipate that bad things are going to happen." Or "My dad left me sitting on a bar stool with a Pepsi while he got drunk. I can't stand to be left waiting." He may recognize why you acted the way you did. "OK, I get why you blew up when I was late the other day."

- Keep humor in your relationship. If you can joke about problems, they won't seem as dire. For example, a young woman blew up at her future spouse at a romantic dinner. "I know what you are thinking," she shouted. "How do you know what I'm thinking?" he asked. "Your nonverbal behavior" she shouted as she stormed out of the restaurant. Her confused fiancé followed her out of the restaurant. "Call me a cab," she ordered. "OK, you're a cab," he answered. She started laughing and returned to the restaurant, where they finished their romantic dinner and she was able to talk about her childhood patterns and how they caused some problems with trust in her adult life.

- Take advantage of your differences. Each of you will have strengths and talents the other lacks. Recognize and utilize these gifts. You are not in competition with one another—you are a team. If one of you is better at decorating, gardening, mechanics, budgeting, expressing feelings, introspecting, or whatever, utilize that person's skills and learn from them. If you can do this, your strength as a couple will be more than the sum of the two of you as individuals.

- Find an older, happily married couple who has dealt with the stresses you are facing in the military and ask them if they will help you succeed in your marriage. Most couples will respond positively to a request of this nature, and they can be invaluable to you if you will bounce decisions off them and follow their suggestions and guidance.

- As mentioned above, seriously consider getting involved with a religion. It is another important aspect in life that you can both share. Most churches and synagogues offer premarital counseling, and this would be of great help to your marriage. Faith in God will give you strength to deal with the stresses you face. Religion provides a moral structure to follow in life. It supports marriage and the family.

Pastors and priests are experienced at helping young couples and can be of great help to you. The fellowship with other sinners who are trying to improve themselves can be a great support. In addition, the church offers structure, guidance, and support for parenting.

- Don't be hesitant to seek professional help. Some individuals (typically male) think asking for help means a person is weak and unable to solve his or her own problems. Some couples think that the time to see a counselor is when you run into serious marital problems. I'm urging you to seek assistance while your relationship is good with the idea of getting some help keeping it good in the future. Think of the counselors, ministers, or older mentors as coaches on your old sports teams. You are new at marriage. These are the pros and they can give you tips and set you on the right path early on in your relationship. The answer is to fix problems early while they are small and prevent major difficulties later on.

- Because one or both of you are in the military, you have some additional stresses.

- You will be required to learn and adapt to the culture of the military organization.

- You will be subjected to frequent geographical moves. You will likely have financial stresses. You will be subjected to prolonged periods of separation, and at least one of you will experience stressful, dangerous assignments overseas while the other functions as a single parent at home. Read this book to help understand and lessen the stresses and adjustments you will both have to make in the military.

Section II: General Considerations

Parenting and Children in the Military

We've discussed the stresses associated with marriage in general with the additional hurdles caused by service in the military. There are about thirty-seven million dependents (spouses and dependent children) of living veterans and survivors of deceased veterans. Together they represent 20 percent of the US population. In 2007 there were over seven hundred thousand children with at least one parent deployed. Thirty-eight percent of active-duty females are mothers. Forty-seven percent of army personnel have children. Seventy-five percent of all reservists, who are older than active duty soldiers, are parents. Having the responsibilities and demands associated with parenthood adds additional stresses for both parents.

Pediatricians have expressed concern recently about the number of drugs being prescribed for the children of parents in the military. This may in part be due to the shortage of mental health professionals available to provide evaluation and counseling for military dependents. Obviously, "military brats" who are dealing with extended separation from a parent and other inherent stresses in the military are more likely to benefit from counseling than medication.

Do not judge yourself on the basis of your children's behavior. In my forty-plus years of psychiatric practice, I've seen great kids come out of what appeared to be terribly dysfunctional families and kids with severe problems who were raised by what appeared to be great parents. There is no guide for perfect parenting. We do the best we can and make mistakes at times. Some of these can be avoided through education and by imitating people who are good parents. Some people say that the measure of a man's success in life is what his children say about him. By that standard, my dad was a great father. My children have always had nice things to say about me, although I know I put time into my work that should have been spent with my oldest daughters over the years. In any event, my four children and one godson seem to be doing well. My grandchildren are all different and all great in their own ways. The suggestions below are not made from my experience as an outstanding parent, but from my observations of what appear to be good parents and their children over years of psychiatric practice.

Here are a few initial suggestions.

- Take parenting classes together. Discuss and agree on your approach to raising children. Some of you will be saying, "We don't have time to read books, seek counseling, and take classes." But you do. Your marriage and your children are top priorities in life, and it is important for them and for you in the future to do everything you can to have a good marriage and to be a good parent.

- I didn't think seminars and classes would have much to offer but, for example, one junior high PTA meeting lecturer said that when your kids want to go to another kid's house, call the parents and see who is going to be there, what is going to be going on, etc. This eliminates your kids being at a party where the parents are away. This prevented lots of problems, although our kids griped about us calling the parents each time.

- Having a child is a great responsibility. To be a good parent you need to make your child your top priority and to provide unconditional love.

- Take care of yourselves and be good role models for your kids. The best thing you can do for your children is to feel good and be happy yourself. When parents are drained but spend time with their children out of guilt, the child thinks, "Mom (or Dad) always seems unhappy around me—I must be a bad person."

Section II: General Considerations

- If your parents did a good job with you, you can use them as role models as you parent your own children at various stages in their development.

- Each stage in your child's life will bring up your own conflicts and difficulties at that same age. (This is one reason why teenagers are so stressful to parents. They remember their own rebelliousness toward their parents, and they don't want their kids to have those angry feelings toward them.)

- Find an older couple who have a good marriage and who seem to be good parents. Ask them if they will serve as mentors to help you be good parents.

- Ask your parents for advice. You may think they had some shortcomings parenting you, but they are older, wiser, and likely to be more patient with their grandkids than they were with you. Bill Cosby's mother was giving money to his children and they were saying how great their grandmother was. Bill said, "That is not my mother—that is an old lady trying to get into heaven."

- Include the children by talking truthfully to them about the family's circumstances and keeping them involved as you prepare for deployment.

- If you think you are running into snags, talk with a chaplain or a professional counselor about the difficulties you are having.

- Be truthful and open with your children.

- Be consistent and dependable. When children know what to expect, they feel secure.

- Home should be a nurturing, secure, loving environment.

- Be cautious about allowing professionals to treat family problems with medication.

In this chapter we've noted the diversity of individuals serving in the military and the impossibility of providing advice for every individual at all times in this book. The recommendation is to take what is helpful for you at each juncture. A few groups were mentioned and their unique stresses described. We noted the frequency of marital problems and divorce among couples where one member is deployed. Because of this we offered advice about making the decision to marry and provided suggestions for enriching the marital relationship. Finally, we made a few comments about parenting.

In the next chapter, I list the main reasons to sign up for the military. I then describe the changes that recruits undergo during basic training (BT) and advanced individual training (AIT). I also describe some of the adjustments spouses and families are forced to make when their loved one becomes a soldier. A positive attitude toward military service and deployment is helpful.

Section III: Predeployment

Chapter One: Induction Changes

Civilian to Soldier

Why did you or your spouse decide to join the military? According to recent surveys of new military recruits, the primary reason given for joining the military is money. Lack of employment opportunity is a current factor. Military pay may not seem that great, but housing, food, rent, medical care, clothing, transportation, equipment, and recreational facilities are free. Combat pay is higher and salaries are tax free while serving in a war zone. The military provides free training and, later on, pays for additional civilian education and training. If one is killed on duty, the person's heirs receive $250,000 in government life insurance payments.

The second reason for joining is patriotism. Many individuals signed up after 9/11 because of the war against terrorism. I've been impressed by the patriotism of the veterans I've gotten to know over the years. They sincerely believe in our country and sacrificing their lives, if need be, in our defense. Dr. Ed Stevenson, the father of McLean Stevenson, star of the *MASH* television series, was a World War I veteran who went to medical school and attempted to enlist in World War II out of patriotism. He reported that every day, as he was going to his office in downtown Bloomington, Indiana, he would run into his aunt and one of her lady friends who would inquire if he had heard from the government. When he answered no, his aunt would say, "I wonder why not." Dr. Stevenson said he got tired of hearing this day in and day out, and so one day when his aunt said, "I wonder why not," he answered, "Well, they aren't taking guys with syphilis." This statement caused his shocked aunt to be silent. A few hours later, his office phone rang and it was his mother. She asked, "Are you getting treatments, Ed?" "For what?" he inquired. "Well, your aunt said you had a venereal disease," she stammered. Dr. Stevenson laughed and said, "I didn't say I had syphilis—I just said they weren't taking men who had it!" (You can see where McLean got his sense of humor!)

Another motivation that is given is because other relatives have served. Here in the Midwest and, certainly in the South, military service is a family tradition. In my own situation, my father and uncle served in the navy in WWII. My cousin was a Marine pilot who did two tours in Vietnam. My father-in-law was in the Bataan Death March and a prisoner of war for 3½ years. Even though the antiwar sentiment of the sixties had begun, when I was told I would be going into the service, I thought it was the natural course of events. I looked forward to receiving the salary and benefits, which were much greater than those I received as a psychiatric resident.

For some, there is the security of a structured, authoritarian organization. Soldiers are told when to get up, when to go to bed, and what to do on a daily basis. Some new troops report that they are looking for the family relationships, structure, and security that the military offers. Some say they haven't decided what vocation they wanted to pursue in life, and time in the military will permit them to decide on their future life course and to gain some maturity. Others report that they are attracted by on-the-job training, educational opportunities, and nondiscrimination. Some say they want to be a part of something larger than themselves. There is still a feeling that the military is part of the initiation into adulthood and that combat is a test of manhood. Some young troops are attracted by the prospect of adventure and excitement of combat.

One Special Forces instructor told me that he asked members of his classes if they had advanced degrees and why they joined the military. Eighty percent had college degrees, and the most common answer was they wanted "to do something" before they settled down with a career.

From what I've observed, the decision to enlist is determined by a combination of these factors. Financial security, patriotism, family tradition, growth, training, adventure, and wanting to make a contribution to society, as well as an attraction to the lifestyle, all appear to be common motivational factors that influence a new recruit's decision to join.

One-third of the military population is made up of minorities. Since the 1960s and Vietnam, the elite social classes do not serve. This causes a dilemma for some troops, who feel that the individuals in the government in Washington, who are making the decisions and ordering them to put their lives on the line, haven't served in combat themselves.

Some recruits are given false promises by recruiters. The recruiter offers the young enlistee a job, money, a means of leaving home, and the promise of adventure, as well as a means of acquiring training and education. These soldiers tell their drill sergeants that the recruiter promised them this or that, to which the DI replies: "He lied." It is probably a good idea to have the recruiter put his promises in writing. Recruiters, anxious to make their quotas, sometimes tell recruits to lie on their applications about their past mental health problems. These often come to light during the stress of military training and result in the individual being discharged for having a fraudulent enlistment or sometimes cause an administrative separation for the service.

In Vietnam I observed that frequently men who wanted to be medics were trained as mechanics while those who wanted to be mechanics ended up as medics. I asked a career officer about this observation, and he said the army wants to train men from scratch and those who think they know something about a particular field are often more difficult to train because they have to first unlearn what they think they know. He said, "There is the right way, the wrong way, and the army way." It is like the famous martial arts story where the young applicant goes to the master to seek training and tells him how much he knows about martial arts. The master silently pours tea into the novice's full cup, causing it to overflow. The surprised young trainee points this out to the master, and the master says, "When your cup is full nothing can be added. To learn you must first empty your cup." This is not as much of a problem in today's volunteer, professional army. Men and women are generally trained in the specialty they choose.

Conversion from civilian to military lifestyle is accomplished in a few weeks during basic combat (BCT) and advance individual training (AIT). Instruction takes on an increased intensity during wartime as both the recruits and the instructors know that the lessons learned will soon be applied in an actual combat situation and the survival of these troops will in large part depend on their training. New soldiers deployed to combat areas in Operation Iraqi Freedom or Operation Enduring Freedom undergo another transformation in the field from newly trained soldier to warrior.

Some critics have referred to the process of entry into the military as brainwashing. Drill instructors admit that they use psychological techniques to manipulate impressionable young recruits

Section III: Predeployment

during the training. The process of degrading the individual and reestablishing him as a group member is similar to a fraternity initiation or joining a gang in civilian life, but it is brought about in a more controlled and professional manner by the experienced drill instructors who utilize years of military tradition and experience. There is the good cop and bad cop pressures of the young drill instructors (DIs) versus the experienced senior DI recruits. Trainees, the majority of whom are teenagers, are confronted with screaming young drill instructors who shout at them that they are "scum," "maggots," and other degrading titles. Corrective training is referred to as "smoking," in which recruits are ordered to do sit-ups, push-ups, low crawl, and other exercises until their muscles fail and they reach a point of physical exhaustion. They are "smoked" at this point. The sergeant asks why they joined. The only correct answer is "To serve our country." Stressful training in adverse environmental conditions forges close friendships and loyalty akin to those that will be later formed in combat. Eventually the relationship to comrades in arms will be stronger than the instinct of self-preservation.

The young men are given buzz haircuts and uniforms. Recruits are housed in barracks together, they eat together in the same mess hall, they share the same shower and toilet facilities, and they train as a group. They may undergo collective punishment for an individual's error. Their individual identities are diminished in importance and are replaced by a group unit identity. It is implicit that the individual's contribution is limited, while the group can accomplish anything. The individual conscience is replaced by the group conscience. Individuals are raised with religious and cultural prohibitions against killing. The group conscience says it is OK to kill if ordered to do so and if the person being killed is an enemy who threatens you, the safety of the country, or your comrades in arms. Just as hand-to-hand combat moves and use of weapons are practiced repeatedly so that they become reflexive, group interaction also becomes so ingrained that members of the unit can anticipate one another's thoughts and actions.

The DIs focus on the recruits making their beds, polishing their brass, organizing their possessions, and cleaning the barracks. In the old days they spit shined their boots but, as CSM Huber points out, today they wear rough-cut boots that are cleaned and not polished. They focus on the details of these tasks and insist on conformity and obedience. They want to keep the conflict with authority at this level so that these men will respond immediately when ordered into battle overseas. Recruits soon learn to respond immediately and without question to orders.

The standards for the physical tests during basic training used to be low enough that the majority of recruits were capable of passing them. CSM Huber says that most recruits today have difficulty passing even these minimal requirements. Trainees are told that by successfully completing the physical training course they have demonstrated that they are exceptional men. This instills pride and a feeling of uniqueness in the group. Military music, flags, and shouted cadence all provide a milieu that emphasizes patriotism and group pride. The bonding that occurs among the men is the most important force sustaining an individual in combat. It is love for fellow soldiers, not hatred for the enemy, that enables warriors to endure the stresses of battle. Concern for the welfare of comrades is a prime motivational factor enabling the soldier to kill the enemy. Killing is condoned as long as the soldier follows the rules of engagement. "Punish the deserving" is the phrase that is used. Honor and fear of appearing cowardly are additional influences that cause an individual to be capable of killing. Men in groups are more likely to shoot at the enemy than they would on their own in the field. Veterans are not murderers, but the idea that the influence of a comrade can cause the individual to act in a way they couldn't on their own was illustrated in Truman Capote's *In Cold Blood*. In this historical fiction, two inadequate ex-cons, Richard Hickock and Perry Smith, killed four innocent family members because of the dynamics of their relationship. It was unlikely that either of them could or would have committed the crime on his own.

Close order drilling was an aspect of training in the eighteenth century, and it facilitated movements and skills associated with loading and reloading muskets. It continues to be a part of basic training in most armies because it instills instantaneous response to orders and esprit de corps. Rifle training "by the numbers" teaches recruits to fire their weapons when ordered. In 1947 Lt. Colonel S. L. A. Marshall wrote a thin book entitled *Men Against Fire: The Problem of Battle Command in Future War.* In it he reported, to the surprise of the military, that only 15 percent of World War II American riflemen in combat fired their weapons at the enemy. Investigation showed that men trained with bull's-eye targets were hesitant to shoot when confronted with live human beings in battle. The military then began to make an effort to condition soldiers to specifically kill the enemy. Military trainers observed that men who fired with a crew were more likely to use their weapons. Seemingly, like Hickock and Smith above, the support of other men and not wanting to appear cowardly in front of comrades enabled them to shoot. Military scientists noted that the more distant and impersonal the situation, the easier for the individual to kill the enemy. Bombers in airplanes who didn't see the targets had little difficulty dropping their killing load on individuals below. Artillerymen and mortar men, who couldn't see their targets, fired their weapons without hesitation. Artillerymen were part of a group and given orders by their superiors. Some gunners did develop psychological problems when they accidentally killed friendly forces. Riflemen who didn't see their targets had fewer difficulties than those who saw their victims. The most difficult situation for most soldiers is close, hand to hand killing with a knife or bayonet. Lt. Colonel David Grossman notes in his book *On Killing* that there is a universal anxiety associated with killing or dying from a bayonet. The army studied the psychological resistances and barriers associated with killing and altered its training methods in order to overcome them. The percentage of men firing their weapons in Korea was 55 percent, and in Vietnam it was 90 percent as the military began training with more lifelike targets. Lieutenant Colonel Grossman noted that men will perform in combat exactly as they are trained. One group of policemen, who were ordered to pick up their brass when they emptied their clips during training, actually stopped during a firefight to pick up their casings! Largely on the basis of Grossman's findings, modern soldiers and police training utilize virtual reality, paint gun, and multiple integrated laser engagement systems (MILES) to make the training as close to actual combat as possible. Nowadays, new recruits are issued weapons early in their training with five blank shells, and they keep one in the chamber. They clear their weapons before entering buildings. This gets them used to having a weapon with them at all times and one that is "loaded" most of the time. Current weapons-training classes utilize weapons that are modified to give a realistic sound, recoil, and muzzle blast simulation. Realistic images of enemy targets as well as friendly targets are projected on a huge screen, and soldiers "fire" their lasers at them. Computers verify bullet strikes. Hundreds of shoot/don't shoot scenarios are presented.

Recruits are taught to respect and obey authority figures. Drill instructors are seen as superiors who are initially hated but soon respected. The senior DI is the recipient of the most respect, while the company commander is seen as a distant godlike figure. It is amazing to see how quickly this phenomenon occurs. I remember driving to Ireland Army Hospital at Fort Knox in 1968 and seeing a new recruit running at full speed across the grounds of the post. He spotted me in the car in my captain's uniform and came to an abrupt halt and saluted me. During the same period, on our psychiatric unit, we had a psychotically depressed, suicidal soldier from Vietnam who was smearing himself with his own feces. When I opened the door to his seclusion room, he snapped to attention and saluted.

During basic training the person's locus of control shifts to subservience to powerful others. Marines are told they can't die without permission. Traits of desensitization, dominance, competitiveness, aggression, compliance, and team bonding are instilled. The soldier responds to authority instantly and, in most cases, without question. In close order drill and rifle practice the young recruit is taught to respond instantly to the commands of his superior. He learns that firing his weapon on command is expected and that killing the enemy is a matter of honor in wartime in the defense of his country and his comrades in arms. Honor is important in the military. To sacrifice oneself for one's comrades in arms is the greatest honor. This is compatible with Christian teachings: "Greater love hath no man than this, that a man lay down his life for his friends" (John 15:13). "He that loseth his life for my sake shall find it" (Matt.10:39). "Whosoever will save his life shall lose it; and whosoever will lose his life for my sake shall find it" (Matt. 16:25). A trainee learns to make decisions based on what is best for the group rather than his own interests. His survival in combat will later depend on his performing by this dictum. Showing cowardice under fire would be great dishonor. This is an important influence to note as it may play a significant role in the current epidemic of suicides among soldiers and veterans.

General George S. Patton set the tone for a macho military attitude toward mental illness during World War II. He was relieved of his command in Sicily for slapping a private suffering from battle fatigue in a hospital tent. He was later quoted as saying, "The greatest weapon against the so-called 'battle fatigue' is ridicule. If soldiers would realize that a large proportion of men allegedly suffering from battle fatigue are really using an easy way out, they would be less sympathetic. If soldiers would make fun of those who begin to show battle fatigue, they would prevent its spread and also save the man who allows himself to malinger by this means from an after-life of humiliation and regret." The heritage of "Blood and Guts" lingers on in the military, and brave men are afraid to admit weakness or to seek mental health assistance. (This resistance to seeking help is a significant factor in the epidemic of suicides among soldiers and veterans today.)

Emperor Napoleon noted that no amount of money would cause a man to risk his life in battle, but he would gladly face his death for a simple piece of ribbon. Personal freedoms and privacy are sacrificed as the individual becomes immersed in the military culture. They may be required to follow rules that make no sense to teach them that their job does not include independent thought or judgment, but rather blind obedience.

Basic trainees are taught to be tough and to deny their feelings. There is a story of the sergeant who lined up his recruits and said, "Pfc. Jones, your mother just died." The private fell to the ground sobbing. The company commander (CO) called in the sergeant and reprimanded him for being so insensitive. "When you have bad news, don't drop it on a fellow that way, lead into the subject gradually," the CO cautioned. The following week the sergeant, cognizant of his commander's advice and the need to be empathetic and tactful, lined up the men. "Everyone with a mother take one step forward—not so fast, Smith." This desensitization and denial can even be seen in the medical field. Medics are caregivers and are perceived as the nurturing members of the military organization, but in a tough manner. For example, during WWII a battalion surgeon stationed on an island in the Pacific noted that the operating room lights in their tents were not bright enough and it was difficult to see what they were doing during surgery. They wired the surgeon general, "We need larger operating room lights."

The surgeon general wired back, "Make bigger incisions." More recently, a Special Forces medic received two Silver Stars and two Purple Hearts for his heroics in the field. He conducted sick call for the unit. Frequently men who were going on patrol developed headaches, backaches, and/or stomachaches the day of the assignment. The medic put two cans of kerosene on each side of the tent flap and put strips of canvas in each can. He would examine a soldier, announce that he was OK and then, as the fellow was leaving the first aid tent, would say, "Take a piece of canvas from each can and wrap it around each of your ankles." "Why?" the soldier asked. "Will that help my backache?" "No," responded the medic. "It will keep the ants from crawling up your legs and eating your candy ass while you are out on patrol." A navy chief petty officer who ran sick call told me how he would put everyone with diarrhea against one wall and everyone with a cough against another wall, and then he would pass out medications. If an individual returned the next day with a cough, he would give them stronger cough medicine. If they returned a third day, he gave them caster oil. "How does that help a cough?" I asked. "They're afraid to," he answered with a twinkle in his eye. I mention these examples to illustrate that nurturing is provided in a tough, macho manner in the service.

Two other examples of this macho orientation in the military occurred at Fort Knox during my tenure there in 1968. A lieutenant was arrested for paying a paperboy to have oral sex with him. It turned out the boy had done the same thing for a number of men on his route, but the commanding general wanted the lieutenant sent to Leavenworth federal prison for life. We admitted him to the psychiatric unit and had him medically boarded out of the army. At about the same time, a sergeant came into the NCO club and was drinking at the bar. He spoke to another sergeant at the bar and asked, "What would you do if your wife was screwing around on you?" "I'd shoot the bitch," the sergeant replied "That's what I thought," said the first sergeant, who then left the bar. A short time later he returned and spoke to the sergeant again. "What would you do with the SOB who has been fucking her?" he queried. "I'd blow him away as well," answered the second sergeant. The sergeant left the bar and returned a short time later. The MPs then arrived and arrested him for murdering his wife and her lover. He did not do any prison time. The military judicial decision was justifiable homicide. In other words, oral sex with a minor deserved a life sentence, according to the general, and double murder was justifiable!

It is said that the military likes to recruit young men and women who cannot conceive of death. Older inductees, who are aware of their mortality and have more responsibilities, tend to be more cautious and concerned with their personal safety. Soldiers learn to isolate their feelings and to deny their fear as part of their initial training. Recruits are taught the precise meaning of military rank and terms. A drill instructor will point out to a trainee that "Yes, sir!" is an inappropriate response to a noncommissioned officer. "You will not address me as 'sir.' I am your sergeant. I work for a living." A recruit who refers to his rifle as "a gun" will be made to run around the post with his rifle in one hand and his other on his crotch, shouting, "This is my rifle, this is my gun, this is for killing, and this is for fun." Military language, in general, is sterile and tends to desensitize the emotional aspects of aggressive behavior. For example, killed in action is referred to as KIA, and wounded in action is WIA. Enemy soldiers are "targets" rather than humans. They are "engaged," "zapped," "blown away," "taken out," "lighted up," instead of being killed. Lieutenant Colonel Grossman feels that the psychological event of killing should be dealt with forthrightly and morally. He notes that some men are opposed to killing but understand the reason they are fighting the enemy and that it is their job to kill if necessary to protect themselves, their comrades, and their loved ones at home. Others kill without giving a second thought.

A small minority of sociopaths enjoy killing and even become addicted to the high associated with taking a life. I heard of a sniper from World War II who became a hit man for the mafia. A Delta friend of mine befriended him on a jump and was surprised years later when the fellow left him the keys to a whorehouse. Apparently, he had no family and no friends closer than this casual acquaintance. I met a ranger in Vietnam who was there for his third tour of duty. He provided several rationalizations as to why he had re-upped for additional tours but finally admitted, "I like killing." One of my veteran pals told me, while high on drugs, that he periodically went to Mexico for trips that were primarily motivated by his desire to kill someone.

For most individuals, however, killing another member of one's own species leads to remorse and guilt. This is significant when it comes to helping veterans deal with their guilt about killing after they return from war. In an excellent article, *The Price of Valor* (*New Yorker.* July 12&19, 2004), Dan Baum reviews the topic of killing and how it has been avoided by mental health workers in the military and VA. My own experience working with veterans causes me to agree with both Lieutenant Colonel Grossman and Baum that guilt about killing their own species causes great suffering for many veterans. I saw a veteran who served as a sniper for seventeen years. He was told to think of his daily mission as a movie and then roll back the film of the "pink clouds" he saw and erase it at the end of each day. He said he did it for years, and it enabled him to go on to the next day's list of targets. After his discharge he said that every target and every "pink cloud" came back to him in his dreams, and he has been haunted by what he did. I've heard many other veterans describe men, women, and children they have killed and how the images of these individuals and the acts of killing them return to them repeatedly in vivid detail. Following orders, impersonal language, and dehumanizing the enemy are all ways to lessen the perception of having killed a living individual. When these defenses break down, most soldiers feel guilt for having taken a life. For example, they sometimes discover personal items on the dead enemy bodies. This causes them to wonder about the details of their victims' lives, what were their families like, who mourned their deaths, and what did they miss in life.

Soldiers in training are introduced to a new language consisting of military terms, abbreviations, and sayings. The new recruit is preoccupied with learning and using this new manner of speaking in an effort to assimilate into the brotherhood of warriors. This is true of every profession. For example, medical students are obsessed with the language and abbreviations of their profession. New psychiatric residents' speech is saturated with the jargon and psychobabble of their specialty. Spouses are frustrated with the novice's preoccupation with the new language and feel excluded.

Recruits identify with their units and with their branch of service. Some had a "meat tag," which is the information from their dog tags (name, Social Security number, blood type, and religion), tattooed on their bodies so that they could be identified if they happened to be blown apart by a mine, IED, VBIED (vehicle-borne IED or car bomb), or enemy shell. They are asked to write a "death letter" to be sent to their loved ones in the event that they are killed in battle. There is a shift of dependence from the family to the combat team.

Recently the army has introduced the concept of BATTLEMIND training. The idea is that the mind, like the body, can be conditioned to withstand the stresses of combat. The acronym stands for:

      B=Buddies (cohesion) vs. Withdrawal
      A=Accountability vs. Controlling
      T= Targeted vs. Inappropriate Aggression
      T- Tactical Awareness vs. Hypervigilance
      L=Lethally Armed vs. Locked and Loaded

E= Emotional Control vs. Detachment
M= Mission Operational Security vs. Secretiveness
I=Individual Responsibility vs. Guilt
N=Nondefensive Driving (Combat) vs. Aggressive Driving
D=Discipline and Ordering vs. Conflict

Each combat trait is accompanied by problems that may stem from it at home postdeployment. These will be discussed in greater detail in the chapter on postdeployment. More recently the training has been referred to as "master resiliency training" (MRT) and has been applied to families as well as soldiers. The military feels that mental fitness should be given the same attention as physical fitness.

Like most trades and professions, there is frequently some humorous initiation of the new individuals. They may be told to "Go find a grid square." (A grid square is the point where longitude and latitude lines intersect on a map.) The hapless recruit asks experienced servicemen, "Do you have a grid square," and are told to go here or there on the post to find one. Some men are sent from unit to unit to pick up a "rifle report."

Our current military relies increasingly on technicality, and this costs money. The night vision equipment, armor plating, and modern weaponry are all expensive. It cost $170 to outfit a soldier in World War II. The current cost is $17,500, and it is estimated the cost could reach $60,000 by the middle of the next decade.

In summary, conversion of a civilian to a soldier results in an individual whose judgment, conscience, and independence are subservient to his group and to military authority. He has forged a close attachment with his unit and his comrades in arms. His identity as an individual is subservient to his membership in the group and he feels that it is logical to sacrifice oneself for the good of his fellow soldiers. Later, in combat, a soldier sometimes develops anxiety problems due to a conflict between his innate will to live and his devotion to duty. Prohibitions against killing are replaced by justification to kill an enemy who threatens the security of his country or his comrades in arms when ordered to do so by his superiors. He has learned to control and suppress his emotions in order to carry out his unit's mission. He strives for honor and abhors cowardice. He respects and instantly obeys military authority. He has been accepted into a band of brothers. He feels a tight interdependent bond to his fellow unit members. His new brothers will have his back in battle, and he will look out for them as well. He uses words, abbreviations, and phrases unique to his new community. These changes and their origins will be important in the future as he strives to reverse the process and go from warrior to soldier and then back to

civilian during the postdeployment phase. There is frequently some hostility felt by warriors for civilians, who, by the warrior's standards, appear to be preoccupied with mundane, self-serving matters. The soldier may think, "Where were you when we were overseas in adverse conditions, in harm's way, fighting for your security at home? Our comrades were sacrificing their own lives for the lives for their fellow soldiers while you are interested only in your own selfish desires."

The military is adept with the psychological methods required to quickly convert civilians to soldiers. Recently the military has developed programs for resiliency training to condition soldiers to endure psychological stress just as they are physically conditioned to bear physical pressures. To date it does not have a similar process to help warriors become soldiers and soldiers return to a civilian lifestyle.

Civilian Family to Military Family

Although the spouses and children did not sign up for the military, they are brought into the military culture along with their husbands and dads. Like their husbands and fathers, they give up many of their constitutional rights as a part of this authoritarian culture. The lack of privacy, subservience to authority, lack of free speech, and, according to the Feres Doctrine, no right take legal action against the military. The military is a tightly controlled, authoritarian system with lack of autonomy and limited privacy where the father is responsible for the conduct of his family. It is a stringent and demanding style of life with frequent uprooting, extended separations, and the possibility of injury or death.

Recruits are young and frequently married. They and their spouses may lack the wisdom and maturity to cope with the adversities they encounter in military life. In the recent past the female spouses were instructed how to dress, and their military husbands were held responsible for their actions. For example, at Fort Knox in 1968, a wife parked in a space labeled "General Officers Parking," thinking that it was for officer parking "in general." Her husband was punished by being required to attend a series of vehicle safety classes and was admonished to instruct his wife on the meaning of parking signs on the post. Wives in the field-grade housing hung out their laundry according to rank. The colonel's wife had priority for the clothesline and was permitted to dry her laundry first. Maintaining a sense of humor is probably the best way to cope with the military. Your life can be happy despite what may appear to be adverse circumstances.

Officers' wives average over forty-one years of age, while enlisted wives average under twenty-five. Wives and children are exposed to the differences in rank among the enlisted, warrant officers, and commissioned officers. They each have different housing, and there is little socialization among them. This carries over to the wives and children as well. These divisions have lessened in recent years. Officers and NCO clubs have been eliminated for the most part. Wives groups now go by first names, and the rank of the spouses isn't mentioned. Frequent changes in assignments affect the families. Wives may have worked their way up to being chairwomen of various committees and charities on the post only to be relocated to a new post where they start at the bottom as new members of the various organizations. Similarly, the children are moved to a new school about every three years and find themselves starting over making friends and proving themselves to a new group of kids. Sometimes this results in joining the less popular group of children, who are an easier group in which to find acceptance. It is difficult for the spouse to find or maintain employment because of the frequent geographical moves. Even when the warrior is home, he or she may be engaged in a mission and be unable to pick up a sick child at school or provide support to his or her employed spouse. Ten percent of married active-duty military personnel were in dual-service marriages.

Wives, like ministers' wives, used to feel their primary job was to support their spouse in his military role. The wife joined groups and behaved in ways that would support and enhance her spouse's military advancement. Current military spouses (and ministers' wives) tend to see their careers as separate from their husband's. In the 1990s over half of military wives were employed.

The concept of honor in the military may be difficult for the spouse to comprehend at first. Many soldiers will sacrifice their own safety and lives for honor. Getting killed is an honorable choice if it is done while carrying out the mission and/or saving the life of a comrade in arms. Cowardice is seen as the worst dishonor. Some warriors feel that their devotion to duty and honor excuses them from responsibilities at home. Military men frequently miss the births of their children because they are deployed or because the mission comes before family responsibilities. It is likely that the civilian husband or wife feels that, unless the spouse was personally strangling bin Laden, he or she should be present for family obligations.

The tendency for men to feel that their activities are more important in order to escape from the chores, and that cooking, cleaning, and child care are "woman's work," is a tradition that goes back thousands of years. On the rocky banks of Cooper's Creek in the Australian Outback are a number of ancient Aboriginal paintings. Our guide, "Desert Dick," told us that no one knew what the symbols meant except that they were sacred and only the men of the tribe were allowed to make them. It dawned on us that the women were back home skinning the kangaroos, feeding the kids, cleaning the camp, and cooking the meals, while the men were lounging on the banks of the creek, probably getting "high" on sacred weed, painting doodles on the rocks—performing their "important religious tasks." Some of this manly heritage of escaping the domestic duties might apply to soldiers and their important military missions. I'm certain that it happens in the field of medicine, where "saving lives" takes precedence over "honey-dos" at home.

As the soldier learns to suppress his feelings, except anger, and avoid any emotional display that might be seen as cowardly by his comrades in arms, he may also try to control the expression of his wife's emotions for the same reasons. One wife complained that her husband would become angry with her when she cried or showed her feelings. She said she tried to comply but found it impossible to do. She also noted that the more successful she was at suppressing her feelings, the less she was able to experience joy or happiness. She discovered that suppression of negative feelings resulted in dampening of positive emotions as well. From a psychiatric standpoint, it would be wise for men to learn from women. We should try to identify and express our feelings. We should also learn to seek help and to let professionals assist us with our difficulties.

The intense bonding between soldiers that is encouraged and developed in the military may cause the soldier to spend time away from home with his or her buddies. The spouse may experience this as less support and attention from the mate. She or he may feel angry at what is perceived as rejection, but it is probably best not to forbid a grown man or woman to do anything. It is best not to try to accompany your spouse while he or she is in advanced individual training. The soldier needs to participate in the bonding encouraged by the military as part of the preparation for deployment and combat later on.

The new soldier is preoccupied with military terms, abbreviations, and jargon, which may be confusing to the spouse and children and cause them to feel more alienated from him and his new group of associates. Wives and/or civilian husbands can learn the acronyms so that they no longer notice them. For example, PX is the post exchange, BDU battle dress uniform, TDY temporary duty, MREs meals ready to eat, NVG night vision goggles, ETS estimated time of separation, OWC officers wives club, NCOWC noncommissioned officers wives club, MOS military occupational specialty, and DEROS date expected to return from overseas. He may use military terms such as Kevlar or jargon like "Vitamin M" (Motrin). You can go to www.milspouse.com and make use of the military spouse glossary of military terms. You can search for a specific term or look through the extensive list in alphabetical order.

In the same way, it is helpful for the wives and civilian husbands to learn the ranks and insignias on the uniforms. It is all part of adapting to a new culture. Each branch has its own jargon, which is even more confusing.

Tongue-in-Cheek Jargon Used by the Three Branches

Here is a contribution by a navy veteran. It illustrates navy and army jargon and pokes fun at the air force. (Everyone envies the air

Section III: Predeployment

force and therefore makes fun of it. In Vietnam we had a sign over the bar that said all air force colonels had to show ID—because they were so young.)

Navy	Army	Air Force
Head	Latrine	Powder Room
Rack	Bunk	Single with Ruffle and Duvet
Mess Deck	Mess Hall/Mess Tent	Dining Facility/The Café
Cookie/Stew	Burner Mess Cook	Contract Chef
Coffee/Mud	Cup of Joe	Vanilla Skim Latte
Bug Juice	Kool-Aid	Shirley Temple
Utilities/Digitals	BDUs/ACUs	Casual Wear
Seaman/Private	Private	Bobby/Jimmy
Chief/Gunny	Sergeant	Bob/Jim
Captain/Skipper	Colonel	Robert/James
Captain's Mast	Article 15	Time-out

61

Supporting You and Your Combat Veteran During and After Deployment

Navy	Army	Air Force
Berthing/	Barracks	BarracksApartment
Skivvies/U-Trau	Underwear	Undies
Thrown in the Brig	Put in Confinement	Grounded
Zoom Bag	Flight Suit	Business
Cover/Head Gear	Beret	Optional
Ship's Store/NEX	PX	Shopping Mall
TAD	TDY	PCS with Family
Cruise/Afloat	Deploy	Huh?
Ground Grabbers	Athletic Shoes	Flip-flops
Die for Your Country	Die for Your Battle Buddy	Die for Air-conditioning
Shipmate/Marine	Battle Buddy	Don't Ask, Don't Tell or Honey
Terminate/Kill	Take Out	Back on Base for Happy Hour
Boon Dockers	Jump Boots	Birkenstocks

Section III: Predeployment

Navy	Army	Air Force
Low Quarters	Low Quarters	Patent Leather Pumps
Seal	SF/Ranger	Librarian
Shore Patrol/	MPs	MPs SF
Ooh-Rah!	Hoo-ah!	Hip-Hip Hurray!
MRE	MRE	Happy Meal to Go
Salute	Salute	Wave
Obstacle Course	Confidence Course	Class 6 Parking Lot
Grinder/Drill	FieldParade Field	What?
Go-Dunk	Snack Bar	Chuck E. Cheese
Pt Test	APFT	"No Conversion Available"
Department of the Navy	DoD	DoD Lite
Midshipman	Cadet	Debutant
Hard-core	Strak	"Way Too Serious"

Spouses should bear in mind that the changes they are experiencing in their mates as they become soldiers will need to be reversed when they return to civilian lives.

Spouses who were aware their mates planned to join the military may not have anticipated how this decision will change the family. Adaptation implies a change in identity for the spouse. It would be helpful to find a spouse who has been happily married to a soldier for a period of time and ask him or her to serve as a mentor. The person could help the new military spouse learn the ropes, including the language and what to expect. Support groups for spouses are available in the military and on Internet websites. These, together with books on the topic, will provide guidance for the new military mate. Veteran spouses who have experienced deployment can provide practical advice for the new spouse facing a mate's hardship assignment.

Hilary Martin, author of *Solo-Ops: A Survival Guide for Military Wives*, notes that the military's supposed interest in wives and family is only lip service because it found that wives don't like being treated as a mere inconvenience and that men don't reenlist if their wives aren't happy. She notes that for wives to survive in the military, they must embrace the fact that it is more than a job—it is a lifestyle change. Wives must expect long periods of separation as part of the military existence. She observes that the military is not family friendly and is not likely to be in the future. She suggests that wives are civilians and are guaranteed free speech under the First Amendment, and she recommends that they gripe away. Martin recommends that the new military wife maintain a sense of humor and adapt to the military lifestyle if she wishes to be happy. The male civilian whose spouse is on active duty is a relatively new phenomenon. Because of the general masculine inability to recognize their own feelings and/or to ask for support, it is even more important for men to take advantage of programs and support available to them in the military.

Obviously the same advice applies to the male spouse married to an active-duty female. It will be a stress for him to support his spouse in the military at home, and more so when she is deployed. He will need to learn the language and customs of the military as well.

> The military has developed a BATTLEMIND acronym for spouses as well.
>
> B=Buddies (Social Support)
> A=Adding/Subtracting Family Rules
> T=Taking Control
> T=Talking It Out
> L=Loyalty and Commitment
> E=Emotional Balance
> M=Mental Health and Readiness
> I=Independence
> N=Navigating the Army (Military) System
> D=Denial of Self (Self-Sacrifice)

Obviously some of these apply as well as to the soldier who needs to talk things out and maintain loyalty and commitment. Emotional balance, mental health, and denial of self can also apply to the warrior. The military recognizes that the mental health of the family is an important psychological influence for the deployed troop's mental health.

Looking Forward to Deployment

Anyone in today's military should anticipate deployment. Activation occurs when the soldier received orders but deployment hasn't started yet. Deployment is a change, not a crisis. Some wives react to activation with shock and feel they are being treated unfairly when their soldier receives orders for deployment. They may ignore the news and act as if it didn't occur. They may think some event will occur that will cause the military to cancel the order, or they may believe that if they are injured or ill their spouse will be excused from going. They may become angry with the spouse for joining the military. They may be upset with the military for deploying people. It's OK to be mad at the military organization, but don't take out your frustrations on your spouse.

Again, joining the military today practically guarantees deployment and repeated hardship assignment. The military forces have been reduced by over one-third in the past decade and yet, with Operation Iraqi Freedom and Operation Enduring Freedom, as well as our other overseas commitments, there has been a 300 percent increase in overseas assignments. A Special Forces NCO recently told me that he knew of one soldier who had been deployed for the eighth time. Deployment is inevitable and part of the commitment that goes with membership in the military. It is important for both the soldier and the dependent spouse to maintain an expectation toward deployment and a positive attitude when orders are received. As the Chinese proverb goes, "It is better to light a candle than to curse the darkness."

Viktor Frankl was a Jewish psychoanalyst who witnessed his family's deaths in a Nazi concentration camp. He decided that the guards could torture him, starve him, or even kill him, but they could not control his attitude. He started doing positive things for his fellow prisoners and cheering them up in the midst of the misery and horrors of the camp. His actions made him feel better and had the effect of making some of the guards feel guilty for their inhumane behavior. He later wrote a book on attitude therapy. Athletic coaches know the importance of attitude. In wrestling they told us to jump up off the mat and act as if we couldn't wait to wrestle another period no matter how tired we felt. This was supposed to have the effect of demoralizing our opponents, but to our surprise it made us feel more energized as well. I told my children when they played tennis in the summer to tell themselves they loved the heat. This also discouraged their opponents and made them feel better as well. My son said he did the same thing while playing football during freezing conditions. In other words, be positive about deployment—it will make you feel better in the long run.

When I received my orders for Vietnam, I had the initial response of getting on my "pity-pot." I attended a meeting in Topeka, Kansas, and showed my orders to one of my professors, Karl Menninger. I thought he would pat me on the shoulder and tell me how sorry he was to see that I had to serve in a combat area. Instead he said, "Wasn't it Thucydides who said: 'War is the father of all things.' Meaning, if you don't get killed, you learn a lot. Many great discoveries come out of military activity." At first I was shocked that Dr. Karl would react to my news in this manner. Later I realized that these were the words I needed to hear. I was, for sure, going to be sent to Vietnam. He gave me good advice. Why not think of the deployment in positive terms? Think of it as an opportunity for adventure, a chance to have unique experiences and learn something about military psychiatry and perhaps combat stress firsthand. My great-uncle, Paul Prehn, was the middleweight wrestling champion of the Allied Armies in World War I. My father and uncle had served in the navy in World War II, my cousin John had done two tours as a marine pilot in Vietnam, and my father-in-law, Wayne Yockey, had been in the Bataan Death March and a prisoner of war in Japan for 3½ years. I would be joining a family fraternity of veterans who served our country in combat. Of course, I was going to miss my family and be apprehensive about the possible dangers of a combat assignment, but there were many positive aspects to the job as well, and, since I was going whether I liked it or not, why not make the best of it? Dr. Karl's seemingly shocking comments had brought me out of self-pity and inspired me to look forward in a positive way to this unique experience!

It is important that soldiers think of deployment in a positive manner. They will be proving themselves as warriors. They will be serving their country and protecting the freedom and safety of their fellow Americans. They will maintain their honor in battle fighting alongside comrades in arms and watching their backs as well. In my opinion, women soldiers have much to gain in terms of their own self-esteem and self-confidence as a result of their military service. They will enjoy a unique experience shared by other veterans of combat. It is for the family at home to view the experience in a positive light and to give that message as well to the departing soldier.

Separation during deployment is stressful and is never easy for even career military wives and husbands. It is difficult to be away from one's mate for an extended period and to worry for his or her safety. The spouse at home will be taking the extra load of acting as both a mother and a father for the children for an extended period. He or she will also be taking on all of the responsibilities for the home during the spouse's absence. One study of 250,000 wives showed that women whose husbands were deployed for eleven months or more had a 24 percent higher rate of depressive symptoms. It also noted that the children of the depressed wives were affected by their mother's symptoms. Nevertheless, the soldier's spouse should try to focus on the positive aspects of deployment. She or he will be supporting an American hero in combat. The spouse will be proving him- or herself by taking on the total responsibility for the family while the warrior is overseas. It is a test of willpower and strength that gives spouses greater self-confidence and self-esteem in the long run. Spouses will find that they are capable of being more independent and self-sufficient than they thought.

Both the soldier and the spouse can talk with the children about deployment. They can encourage them to be proud of their father who is serving his country overseas to protect the safety and freedom of their fellow Americans. Children, particularly younger children, are likely to be more open with their negative feelings and express their fear for their father's safety and anger at his prolonged absence from the family. When I told my six-year-old daughter, Cathy, about my impending departure for Vietnam, she asked, "Are you going to get shot?" It is important to try to answer the children's questions simply and honestly and to learn from their open emotions. But parents should avoid information that might cause undue anxiety for the child. There is unspoken anxiety and anger between the parents that is inhibited by concern for one another. Soldiers tend to feel anger toward anyone who has a safer, more comfortable assignment then they do (the rear echelon motherfucks, or REMFs). They would never express these negative feelings toward their loving spouses, who are about to look after the home and family alone while they are away. The future warrior feels apprehension about the unknown combat assignment, but training as a soldier causes him to suppress feelings of fear. Similarly, the waiting wives or husbands may be angry at having all of the family demands and responsibilities foisted on them for a year. Some spouses feel as though they are being given all the demands and responsibilities while their soldier goes off with his or her buddies and receives all the attention and glory. The waiting spouses are frightened for their mates' safety, but the soldiers discourage the expression of their feelings. The waiting spouse feels anger and fear but doesn't want to vent these feelings toward an American hero who is serving his or her country and who might be injured or killed. The children's direct expression of their fears and frustrations may lead to a more open discussion of these feelings between the spouses.

We've described acceptance of deployment by the soldier and the spouse and how things go better if they both maintain a positive relationship. This is not to minimize the anxiety that they both will likely experience. During Vietnam we had some drafted soldiers who were handcuffed to their plane seats in order to get them overseas. Some conscientious objectors would say, "You can make me go to Vietnam, but you can't make me shoot my weapon." The sergeants would reply, "That's OK, you might stop a bullet for a good man." Today's soldiers are volunteers, better trained and, in most cases, better motivated. Nevertheless, I learned from some of my Special Forces friends that a number of their experienced, well-trained NCOs developed psychosomatic complaints and tried to get out of going overseas when they received orders. They looked good working and receiving the benefits of their stateside assignments but couldn't face the prospect of going to war. The sergeants said they were pleasantly surprised to find other men rise to the occasion and fill the positions vacated by those who avoided deployment.

New recruits are changed by the training they receive on entering the military.

It is important that they and their spouse recognize the changes taking place and how they affect their relationship. If one person in a relationship changes, the other one has to change as well. Recognizing this fact and learning to adapt to the military culture will facilitate the couple's adjustment in the long run. Deployment is a fact of life in today's military. Couples entering the military today should recognize this and anticipate that they will be separated for an extended period of time. Anticipation and planning can lessen the stress of deployment.

In this chapter we've noted the motivations for joining the military. We then described the changes men undergo during basic and advanced military training. Haircuts, uniforms, a new language, strenuous training as a group, punishment of the group for the failings of the individual, intimidation, and appeal to patriotism are all influences that melt the individual into becoming a member of a group. Individual thought and initiative are subverted to that of the organization and the group to the extent that men may sacrifice their own lives for the welfare of their comrades and are trained to kill under specific rules of engagement, when ordered to do so, and in self-defense and the defense of their fellow soldiers. They learn to suppress their feelings and focus their anger.

The family learns that the mission and unit ties often come before the needs of the family. They learn to adapt to the military community, its language, and its customs. Loved ones must adjust to the long hours, absences from home, financial stresses, and frequent relocations that are a part of military life. Both the soldier and the family have to deal with their fear of combat and extended separation. It is important to remember the early changes that the individual went through going from civilian to soldier and that the family went through adjusting to the military, because some of them may get in the way when the warrior and the family try to readjust to civilian life after deployment.

In the next chapter we will discuss some of the concrete steps that soldiers and their families can take to prepare for the hardship tour.

Section III: Predeployment

Chapter Two: Advance Preparation for Deployment

Everyone joining the military today should anticipate and plan for deployment. It is never too early to prepare. There may be a tendency to procrastinate and hope that your soldier will not receive orders. You may find yourself thinking that, in some magical manner, you will be spared this stress. It is, in my opinion, better to assume that he or she will be deployed and to begin to make your plans and arrangements for a period of separation early on. These plans will, first of all, include organizing the concrete arrangements you will need to make regarding your housing arrangements, legal and financial considerations, your car, medical problems, child care, and schooling. Next, you will want to have in-depth discussions regarding effects of separation on your relationship and with the children. Part of these talks will be ideas to reduce the stresses for all concerned and how to preserve and strengthen the loving family bonds while you are apart. Finally, you will want to explore the psychological effects of deployment on each of you and to identify some of the feelings you may each have about this situation. Psychological preparation is as important as physical conditioning.

Concrete Preparation for Deployment

In this book I won't provide detailed checklists for the soldier and the spouse to follow as they prepare for deployment. These are available on the Internet and in several books. One particularly good resource is *Surviving Deployment: A Guide for Military Families* by Karen M. Pavlicin. This book has useful lists to help prepare for deployment. They are thorough and are easily located by typing "deployment checklists" in your computer search engine.

We will discuss, in general, some of the ideas the soldier and spouse need to consider as they get ready for deployment.

Home and Automobile Repairs

It is a good idea to take an inventory of repairs that need to be done and to carry them out before deployment. Have a list of repairmen to call if things break down during deployment.

Legal and Financial Items

Make sure you have a current will prepared. Have a file with copies of all-important documents available for your spouse (birth certificate, living will, medical insurance, orders for deployment, ID cards, titles, etc.). The government thrives on paperwork. During World War II a soldier was stationed on a remote island in the Pacific. He was bored out of his mind. He decided, as a joke, to create a form that resembled the hundreds he received and titled it "Fly Report." He counted the number of flies stuck to the flypaper in his office and recorded the number for each day. Each month he submitted his "Fly Report" to the surgeon general's office in Washington, thinking they would get a kick out of his tongue-in-cheek spoof of military paperwork. To his surprise he discovered that the surgeon general wired all of the other island stations in the Pacific demanding to know why they had failed to submit their Fly Reports. This is a true story of how ridiculous the government paperwork has become. You do need the proper form to get anything done in the military. See to it that the nondeploying spouse has power of attorney and that her name is on all accounts so that she will have access to them. Let her know the sources of income that will be available and when to expect the checks. Arrange for direct deposit of your paycheck for your spouse. List the monthly expenses and arrange for automatic payment of regularly reoccurring bills. Provide a list of credit card numbers, your Social Security number, and important phone numbers she might need. The two of you should sit down together and prepare a budget she can follow during deployment. Keep a file of paid bills.

Housing

You and your spouse will need to discuss where the family will reside while you are deployed. Locating near the post will offer the advantage of having the support of other wives whose spouses are deployed and access to the post facilities (commissary, medical, etc.). On the other hand, many spouses opt to be near their families for their support and help with the children. Once a decision has been made, the couple can begin to plan for a place to rent or purchase, questions of maintenance, insurance, security, location of schools, babysitters, day care, shopping facilities, transportation, and, if the spouse plans to work, job opportunities. Bills for rent, insurance, water, gas, telephone, electricity, and waste/trash services can be automatically paid.

Mundane matters such as the phone numbers of repairmen (plumber, furnace and air-conditioning, electrician, cable or satellite television company, and general handyman) can be recorded. Locate the fuse box, find where to shut off the water, learn how to change the furnace filter, and locate the pilot lights on the furnace and water heater. Record emergency numbers and agencies that might be needed (Red Cross, military ombudsman, insurance agent, etc.). Make duplicate keys for the house. Consider a security system.

A home tool kit is helpful. Spare lightbulbs, filters, toilet plunger, flashlight, first aid kit, and extension cords are handy to have.

Transportation

Make sure registration, insurance, and taxes are up-to-date during deployment. Service on the vehicle should be up-to-date and the spouse should have the number and location of the facility to turn to for service if needed. It is a good idea to have duplicate keys for the vehicle.

Communication

Have a list of phone numbers of friends and family and provide them with the addresses and means to contact the deployed serviceman. Talk about the contact of your communications in advance. It is probably best not to try to solve problems or share negative news long distance. The warrior doesn't want to be distracted from his or her focus on the mission, and you don't want to hear things that will aggravate your fears for your soldier's safety. Start thinking ahead and provide your warrior with addressed envelopes and postcards to make it easy for him or her to send you snail mail on a regular basis. Get two tape recorders and pack one and lots of tapes for your warrior so you can exchange verbal messages to one another. Videotape your warrior reading bedtime stories to the kids. Take pictures of the warrior with you and with the children to post at home. Send lots of pictures of you and the kids with the warrior. If you each have laptops, talk about how you are going to communicate by e-mail. For example, websites and e-mails may not be that confidential. You might want to pack a journal for your warrior where he or she can keep track of daily events, thoughts, and feelings to share with you postdeployment. You may want to keep your own journal for them to look at postdeployment to help him or her understand your year on your own.

Section III: Predeployment

Command Sergeant Huber, a Vietnam veteran who has a son-in-law who has been serving at the "tip of the sword" in combat areas around the world, made the following comments about communication today.

With respect to your book and the issues of those serving in combat areas since Desert Storm One, one area I believe is significantly different from our time in Vietnam is the almost instantaneous telecommunications available between warrior and family. And while this is seen as a benefit by most, it puts tremendous stresses on both the warrior and the spouse or significant other; most warriors do not want to burden their families with the risks they face, nor can they for reasons of operational security or for the safety of their families (especially so for those in Special Operator community). So while Skype and other VOIP services can help the warrior stay in touch, additional stressors come into play if the family does not fully appreciate and understand their role as the warrior's support team rather than as the dependent. The warrior also faces the stress of not being open and honest with family as he limits or hides the facts of the risks he faces (for reasons of operational security) while communicating in a video teleconference.

As a Military Affiliate Radio System phone patch operator providing stateside telephone calls for soldiers during Desert Storm One and later for those in Somalia (Blackhawk Down), I've had the deployed army radio operator give me (an active CSM) an unofficial current local threat brief or tactical situation during the period when the phone numbers and calling parties were being exchanged, requesting that information not be released to the called parties; I've then observed one soldier after another tell family members or friends that any news of fighting, rockets, mortars, or bombings "are miles away" when in fact they were not.

Further I've had family members who have been members of the special operator community who have shared with me that their spouse does not know what they do or what they have experienced; this has been validated on numerous occasions when I have asked the spouse about one situation or another and have received a reply that she has not been told for her own protection.

I've wondered whether the current capability of instant, face-to-face communication between home and warriors is positive or negative. It makes it harder for the soldier to detach and focus on the job at hand. It would seem to me to make soldiers more concerned for their personal safety. On the other hand, it would maintain a stronger bond between the warrior and his loved ones at home.

Medical

Have medical insurance cards available and copies of medical records for the spouse and children. Have a list of emergency and routine numbers of medical providers and pharmacies, as well as a list of medications taken regularly and of children's immunizations.

Overseas

The soldier may want to take an iPod with favorite music to help pass periods of loneliness and boredom. A laptop will help with communication and sending pictures. A flash memory stick to store pictures and a digital camera will help him obtain, store, and send photos to let the family know what his life is like.

Maintaining Healthy Relationships between the Soldier and the Family during Deployment

The prospect of a lengthy separation, the hardship conditions and possible dangers for the soldier, the increased demands on the waiting spouse, and the absence of a parent for the children is a traumatic, shocking, and painful situation to contemplate. A 1994 survey of service families revealed that 46 percent of the couples said that separations are a chronic source of high stress. Couples going through multiple deployments report that the process becomes more difficult and stressful. The soldier, because of his training to suppress feelings, may discourage the expression of emotions by the spouse. The waiting spouse may shut down, and they may detach from one another to lessen the immediate pain of separation. Some couples fill up their time with busywork to avoid thinking or feeling about the impending departure. Some distance themselves and avoid one another to avoid uncomfortable feelings. Others cling to each other, trying to store up their time together. Some get angry with their spouse to make it easier to leave them and to push them away. Some try to be cold and professional. It is better to discuss the shock and painful contemplation of deployment. It is important for couples to reaffirm their love for one another and to reassure each other that they will be thinking and loving the other for the entire time that they are apart. It's important for the soldier to be kind, gentle, and patient with his spouse. Don't treat her like a one-night stand. Cut back on your social obligations for the time preceding your departure and devote time and love to your spouse and children. It isn't unusual for couples to wonder if this will be the last time they will see one another. They worry if things will be the same when the soldier returns home (they won't be).

Soldiers should tell their spouses that they recognize the extra burdens they have and that they appreciate what they will be doing while they are away. Give her or him a romantic card. Hide little gifts around the house for her or him. Ask for photographs of her or him to take with you. Give her or him flowers (most guys like the thought behind the flowers whether they admit it or not).

It would be helpful to discuss and agree upon some rules for communication during deployment. The soldier should recognize that his or her spouse will be alone at home with more than twice the ordinary demands as she or he assumes both parental roles and the entire responsibility for the home and finances. She or he may take on an outside job as well. Waiting spouses are going to be worried for their warriors' safety while they are deployed. It would be best if the warrior did not relate any information that might cause those at home undue concern. If he is exposed to danger or some friends are killed or wounded, the warrior should not discuss these negative events with his wife while he is deployed. Later, after the veteran returns home, he may want to share what the year was like, but only when the loved ones can see that the veteran is safe. In the same way, it would be best for the waiting spouse to avoid bringing up topics that might cause concern for the soldier overseas. If the situation is one that the warrior has no control over and is something that might cause concern or worry, it would be best not to raise the issue.

Trust issues and fidelity are major concerns during deployment. Sixty-two percent of the first marriages of combat veterans end up in divorce. It would be helpful to reassure each other that they love only their partner and that each will be faithful to the other while they are apart. Infidelity causes major problems in a relationship and frequently leads to divorce. Even when the couple remains together, there are wounds to their relationship that remain indefinitely. If one or the other of you has something to confess, do it to the chaplain and not to your spouse.

E-mail and satellite phone contact didn't become common until the late 1990s. Communication in Vietnam was slow (snail mail or MARs calls, which were patched together voluntarily by a group of ham radio operators). As a result, soldiers in Vietnam detached from "the world" and focused on their jobs in country until they became short and the fact that they might make it home alive dawned on them. When this occurred they became concerned for their personal safety and were reluctant to leave the base camp, go on patrols, or take risky assignments.

Preparing Children for Deployment

Both the father and mother should talk to the children about deployment. They can be upbeat about the father or mother serving his or her country and defending the folks back home. Departing parents need to tell the children how much they hate to be away from them, how much they will miss them, and how they will be thinking of them and sending their love and kisses daily while they are away. In the discussion they should be truthful but minimize the dangers involved. If a child is restless, moody, or unmanageable, this is likely a sign of being unable to express negative feelings of anxiety, depression, or anger directly. Brief teachers, principals, school nurses, and school counselors about the deployment so that they can keep an eye on the children for any changes in behavior. Let the professionals know how sensitive the children will be to negative comments about the war.

Younger children may not remember the deployed parent on his or her return. Older children may withdraw, and teens may rebel against any change in rules or a returning authority figure.

Some families have a bowl of candy with the same number of pieces as the days the deployed parent has to serve overseas. The children can take a piece each day and have a concrete way of seeing how long it will be until the parent returns. Some families draw a timeline on a poster on the wall and keep track until Dad or Mom returns. Show the children a map of where the parent will be serving and talk about the environment he will be living and working in overseas. The father or mother could have the children draw pictures that he or she could take on deployment. Toddlers may not remember the deploying parent. Pictures of the infant with the soldier can be referred to during deployment to remind the toddler of the absent parent. The parent could videotape himself reading stories, and the kids could watch and listen to the tapes during the parent's absence. Take a picture of each child with the deploying parent. Record him or her singing lullabies to the children. Buy two tape recorders so you can mail tapes back and forth.

Take pictures of the departing warrior doing normal things alone and with each of the kids and put together an album that the kids can look at during deployment to remember how he (or she) typically was around the house and with them.

It is helpful to set up a consistent routine for the children at home. Children crave the stability of routine. Be honest in conversations and be prepared for them to ask about people dying overseas. They may want to know what the family will do if Dad doesn't return. The military has a CD-ROM called *Your Buddy C.J.* that has games with a bear in a red T-shirt who talks about being upset about a parent who was going to leave. "Now I don't know what to think—I'm really sad."

Children are more open and honest than adults and are likely to express their anger at being left, their fears for their father's safety, and their sadness at being away from him for a year. Have the children help the departing parent pack. Make sure the children see the parent leave. After Dad or Mom leaves, take the kids to do something fun rather than bring them home to an empty house.

Parents should remember that taking care of yourself is probably the best thing you can do for the children. If you are rested, happy, and secure you will convey this to the children, who are sensitive to your feelings. This will make them feel happy and secure as well. To help yourself, think of yourself as a tree. The more roots a tree has the better able it is to weather storms. In the same way, the more sources of gratification and support you have during deployment the more secure you will be in the face of the increased demands and stresses you will be facing. Enlist the help of family, friends, and experienced spouses who have been through deployment. Make use of the government-sponsored support groups and agencies that are available. Turn to your minister, chaplain, or priest for help. Utilize professional mental health services. This advice is more likely to be followed by a waiting wife than a waiting husband because of the male tendency to try to solve problems himself, his inability to recognize his feelings or express them, and his resistance to asking others for assistance. It is important that waiting husbands recognize these shortcomings in themselves and strive to overcome them. Developing a support system, talking with others about your stresses, and letting others help you will greatly ease your time of separation from your spouse.

Psychological Aspects of Deployment

The orders for deployment frequently precipitate what was described by Laurie B. Lone, PhD, and Matthew J. Friedman, MD, PhD, in their book *After the War Zone: A Practical Guide for Returning Troops and Their Families* as "anticipatory grief" in which the spouse begins to experience the loss of the soldier before he or she has actually departed. The psychological process of deployment is similar to mourning. In this case it is an ambiguous loss in which the soldier is still alive and walking around but is not emotionally available to the spouse or the family. He or she, in turn, experiences an ambiguous loss of the spouse and children who are emotionally unavailable. The stages of mourning during deployment are anticipatory grief where both parties are still together but are psychologically imagining and experiencing separation in their minds; shock, with many spouses reporting being initially dazed and disoriented when they begin to accept the reality of their impending separation; and next a feeling of sadness and depression. The couple may become clingy and try to be together constantly during this period, but more often they get busy and pull away from one another in an effort to avoid the pain of parting. The spouse feels as though everything is an effort, cannot experience joy, withdraws from social contacts, has difficulty making decisions, and ruminates about negative topics. Next the spouse may become irritable and feel that she or he and the spouse have been treated unfairly by the military. He or she may express rage toward the spouse for joining the military, his or her acceptance of the deployment, and for leaving the waiting spouse with all the responsibilities for the children and for home. It isn't unusual for the spouse at home to feel the deployed spouse gets to hang out with his or her buddies and avoid the demands and responsibilities at home. The soldier goes through a mourning process as well. He or she may feel irritation at the spouse's anger. He may think that the spouse is going to be home safe and sound while he is overseas in adverse conditions risking his life for his country.

Soldiers in combat tend to be angry with those behind them who have safer, more comfortable assignments. This extends back to civilians at home. Complaining about little problems at home is irritating to warriors who have seen their buddies killed or wounded and who are facing death on a nearly daily basis themselves. The adverse climatic conditions, primitive living accommodations, separation from home, and fears of death and injury all cause your warrior to be quick to anger. You may feel that he is with his buddies while you are isolated among civilians. He has a job to do while you've taken on the jobs of both parents at home. You are lonely and frustrated but have to be positive and supportive for the warrior and the children. All these factors may cause you to be short tempered as well.

When I was a psychiatric resident at the Menninger Clinic, the average stay for a hospitalized patient was one year. We saw our inpatients daily, and over the lengthy period we cared for them they developed intense feelings (transference) toward us. Whenever we scheduled a vacation, we would begin preparing our patients by talking to them a month before we were due to leave. Every day we would ask them about their feelings about our leaving. They would become increasingly irritated and ask if we thought we were that important. They would object to our seeming preoccupation with this topic and say they were glad we were going but tired of hearing about it. Some would caution us that we might be killed by a tornado or accident while we were gone. Those patients who were able to express their anger about out departure were able to adjust to the covering doctor during our absence with little upset. Those who failed to do so took out their anger on the hapless resident who was taking over while the patient's doctor was away. If the future waiting spouse is able to express anger about the soldier's leaving the waiting spouse with the full load of the children and the home, it will be easier for him or her while the soldier is away. Similarly, if the soldier is able to verbalize irritation toward those who remain in safer, more comfortable surroundings, his or her adjustment will be easier as well. The soldier should recognize the changes he or she will undergo while away and remember that the family will be changing as well. It is unrealistic to think things will be the same when he or she returns. Change is certain and discussion of the experiences and changes as well as adjustment to them will be the theme of the postdeployment period.

Relational Aspects of Deployment

The two of you may have the tendency to withdraw from one another to lessen the impending pain of separation. Try to avoid the tendency to pull back from the relationship. Talk about how painful it feels to contemplate being apart for an extended period and your fears for each other's welfare during that time. Spend as much time together as a couple and as a family as possible. Store up some positive memories you can all think about while you are apart. Talk about the upcoming deployment and share how you feel about it and about one another.

It is normal for each of you to experience anger. Talk about your frustration with the situation and the extra burdens you each will have during your year apart. Anticipate the adjustments you will have to make to each other after an extended period of separation.

Start Preparing a Support System

The warrior will have lots of support from comrades in arms who are in the same situation. The spouse at home will need to muster his or her own support system. The military has a number of organizations for waiting wives and husbands as well as children. If you are planning to be away from a military post, you may need to look elsewhere. It may be possible to make contact with some of the military support groups by e-mail. Of course family members can be enlisted if they are nearby. Close friends can be contacted and asked for their help. If there are other spouses in the same boat, contact them for mutual support. Get on the Internet and hook up with other waiting spouses and others who have interests in common with you. Think of yourself as a tree. A tree with one root is vulnerable if something happens to that source of nurturance. To strengthen yourself and prepare for the adverse conditions you will be facing, try to establish as many sources of support and assistance as you are able to develop. These are people you can call on in times of need. They are friends who are positive and will cheer you up when you are down. They are individuals who can spell you with the children and your household duties so that you can get away and recharge when you need to do so. You may have some you can vent to and express your frustration and anger when you need to do so. These are friends who have good marriages and who understand the stresses you face in the military and can help you cope with them. You may include professionals you can turn to for advice, support, and nonjudgmental listening.

Forming a supportive network may be easier for female spouses than for men, but it is no less important that a man who is taking care of the home fires make the effort to develop friendships and professional contacts to help him get through this arduous time of separation and worry.

Upcoming Schedule

Serving as both parents, looking after the house and car, and possibly working will keep you occupied, but you need to be thinking about sports, hobbies, classes, and perhaps something you wouldn't be able to do if your warrior was not deployed. Line up some activities for yourself and for your children to fill your schedule. Make sure some of the events are gratifying and fun for you. Pay attention to your diet and exercise, as your state of health will affect the way you cope with stress. Get up and get dressed each morning and pay attention to your appearance. Looking good helps you feel good. Make sure you are eating healthy foods, getting regular exercise, and seeing the doctor on a regular basis. Your health and appearance are important factors in your ability to cope with stress during deployment. A regular schedule is important for the children and for you as well.

In the next section we will discuss the conversion of the new soldier to a warrior that occurs in the war zone during deployment. He or she will reinforce the lessons received in basic and AIT. He or she will be initiated into a unit and form tight bonds with comrades in arms. His or her focus will be on the mission. He or she will avoid conveying any news that might cause the folks at home to worry for his or her safety. Meanwhile at home the spouse will take on the responsibilities of being a single parent, manage the household, and possibly work outside the home as well. She/he will be praying for the warrior's safety and trying to boost his/her morale while keeping any news of stress at home away from him/her so that he/she can focus on the mission.

IV: Deployment

Chapter Three: Soldier to Warrior, Spouse to Military Waiting Spouse

Soldier to Warrior

Entry into the military begins with a hell week in basic training and is similar in many ways to fraternity hazing, a primitive tribe's rite of passage into manhood, or a gang's initiation of a new member. Women entering the service have, in addition, the adjustment of living and training in a predominately male environment. Entering the combat zone and the transition from soldier to warrior takes place in a similar but less formalized manner. The FNG (fucking new guy) is initiated into his new combat unit by being confronted with his or her worst fears. Entering Vietnam was, to me, like walking through the looking glass in *Alice in Wonderland* and entering a parallel existence.

When I first went to Vietnam, the pilot of the commercial plane that flew us into Bien Hoa was ex-military. He took it upon himself to tell us "war stories" over the intercom as we approached the airport. He described how they received fire when they landed in country in the past. On my second flight to Vietnam (I went home on a TDY assignment to testify at a murder trial) I sat next to a ranger who showed me pictures of pigs eating dead NVA soldiers, apparently in an effort to gross me out.

When we deplaned in Vietnam, we initially felt as though we were walking into an oven. We immediately began to perspire. A planeload of men who had completed their year's tour were waiting in two lines to take our "freedom bird" back to the world. They hooted and jeered at us as we trudged heads down, dripping with sweat, and giving off shit-eating grins (SEGs) through the gauntlet of combat veterans. "Here come the FNGs," they shouted. "Kill yourself now. You're going home in a body bag. Only 365 days to go," they yelled. At our units, our informal initiation and what we referred to as "pimping" continued. The fellows who picked me up at the replacement station to go to the First Infantry Division later told me they had conspired to try to increase my anxiety. They arrived with M-16s, flak jackets, and helmets and told me war stories all the way to the division.

Things haven't changed that much over the years, except currently men typically go to combat with their units or combat teams. This facilitates their adjustment by having the support of comrades they've known and trained with in the States. Veterans who are getting close to leaving country teach new men the ropes. The tradition of relating "war stories" and initiating the FNGs continues. It seems to me that women veterans tend to be more supportive to new arrivals than men, and there is less of the "pimping" seen among men (which is a mechanism developed by preadolescent boys to help one another cope with stress).

Hypervigilance

No one has to teach the FNGs to be hypervigilant—they just are. When you land in a combat zone your adrenaline is flowing, you are naturally on the alert, and everyone looks threatening. On the way to the division in Vietnam, local field workers wearing black pajamas looked like Vietcong (VC) to me. Later in my tour, the same route and people appeared peaceful and friendly. I had a similar experience when my junior high daughter, Cathy, and I were separated from our tour group in a casbah. I suddenly became hyperalert, and everyone I saw looked as if they would be happy to slit our throats and take our passports. I explained to one of them that we were lost, and he took us back to our hotel and gave us an individual tour on the way. He turned out to be a very friendly fellow and a gracious host. Just like in Nam, my perceptions shifted and the place went from scary and threatening to friendly and interesting in some areas. In new, unfamiliar locations, the hypervigilance returned and remained. Vietnamese teenagers on mopeds, called "cowboys" in Saigon, for example, were known to toss grenades onto jeeps or put them into gas tanks. We waved our weapons and yelled "di di" at them to keep them at a distance from our vehicles. Soldiers in OIF and OEF maintain their watchfulness because of suicide bombers, IEDs, and VBIEDs.

My Big Red One escorts dropped me off in front of the docs that first day in the division. The physicians had their own form of initiation. The docs sat in their skivvies in their lawn chairs and interviewed sweating FNGs by asking them intimate sexual questions and observing how they responded. I grossed some of them out by telling them my name was Colonel Lingus. Each unit had its own way of greeting FNGs. The pilots would host a party for their new men and then, once they were sufficiently drunk, stand them on a table and the unit would sing to them (to the tune of "Camptown Races"):

"You're going home in a body bag, doo dah, doo dah
You're going home in a body bag, oh dah doo dah day.
Shot between the eyes, shot between the legs,
You're going home in a body bag, oh dah doo dah day!"

Suppression of Feelings

These informal greetings confront new soldiers with their worst fears and are what behavioral psychologists would call "flooding." Once we were hit in the face and "flooded" with the things that most frightened us, we stopped being so anxious and figured we could do whatever these guys could do. The other guys were alive and well, and so why be nervous? It reinforced our tendencies to suppress our feelings and to "pimp" one another. For example, in the medical battalion the newest doctor got the next assignment. Captain Ross Guarino was our company commander, and Bob Anzinger was our newest doctor. Ross walked up to Anzinger after lunch and told him the policy of giving the latest assignment to the newest doctor and that he was it. Bob asked what the assignment was, and Guarino said it didn't look good. An infantry unit had requested a doctor, and its landing zone (LZ) was too hot to land the helicopter and so Anzinger would have to be inserted by cable, probably under fire, to reach the unit. All the docs left the mess hall with Anzinger and stood around quietly as he packed his duffle bag. He looked scared and as if he was about to cry. The tension was thick as the doctors stood thinking they felt sorry for Bob but were glad they hadn't been given this assignment. Finally I said, "Bob." Everyone looked up, thinking the psychiatrist would know the right words to say. "Yeah?" he answered. "If anything happens to you, can I have your Nikon?" "What!" he exclaimed. "You SOB!" But then he began laughing, which broke the tension, and the other docs joined in. This is the type of "pimping" that helped us survive. If a doc was going on rest and recuperation (R&R) leave, the others would tell stories of planes that crashed or guys who were ambushed on the way to their R&Rs. When a fellow returned from R&R, the other guys "forgot" his name and talked about how great things were during his absence. The fellow about to leave at the end of his tour would have a party for those who remained and give them his things while lamenting the fact that he would now have to eat steaks, drink drinks without iodine, be given exposure to air-conditioning, use flush toilets, and that sex would probably be forced upon him at home. He might add that he would now have to miss the Bob Hope show at Christmas.

These rituals and "flooding" by the veterans help the FNGs to adapt to their new assignments. They learn to further suppress their feelings and engage in the counterphobic pimping of their warrior brothers in arms. Soon those who are actual combatants will prove themselves further by their conduct in the field. Those who serve outside the wire will conduct themselves with honor and bravery and prove that they are courageous. Those in supporting rolls deal with the chronic stress of boredom interspersed with brief periods of sheer terror. Never knowing when a suicide bomber, IED, VBIED, mortar, or rocket may go off leads to a chronic state of tension.

Emotional Detachment

The new guys imitate the scatological language of the combat veterans. In Vietnam we used the *f* word so many times we put it between syllables (fan-fucking-tastic, un-fucking-believable). The Vietnam veteran soldiers told us they had two theories as to how we could win the war. Someone had taken the amount of money expended on the war and divided it into the number of NVA killed and figured it cost us $75,000 per NVA soldier. The plan was to fly around Vietnam with bags containing $50,000 in quarters. Every time a Vietnamese was spotted we would drop a bag on them. If it hit them it would kill them and we would save $25,000. If we missed they would take the money and retire—either way we eliminated a Vietnamese soldier at a cost savings of $25,000. Another solution was to put all the friendly Vietnamese on ships, kill all the remaining Vietnamese in country, and then sink the ships. One test that was advocated was to point your rifle at any Vietnamese you spotted. If they ran, they were Vietcong (VC) and you should shoot them. If they didn't run, they were well-disciplined VC and you should shoot them. Vietnamese were referred to as "dinks," "slopes," and sometimes "gooks." They referred us to as "long noses." In OIF and OEF, Afghanis and Iraqis are referred to as "hajjis" and "towel heads." Their habit of shouting "Allahu Akbar" when shooting was referred to as "pray and spray" by our troops.

Degrading labels for the enemy are ways to dehumanize them, which makes it easier to accept their deaths. The jokes about killing them relieve the anxiety that accompanies taking another person's life. As the soldiers learn to become warriors, their tendency to suppress their feelings is reinforced. They dehumanize the enemy and desensitize themselves to facilitate killing them. They relieve their guilt and tension through humor. In the field their ability to kill the enemy is augmented by the presence of their comrades in arms. They want to watch their backs and distinguish themselves as brave, honorable men. Modern warfare involves fighting insurgents and winning the hearts and minds of the local inhabitants. The Russians ignored the latter aspect of guerrilla warfare and lost because the natives turned against them and supported the Taliban. We understand the need to engender local support for our efforts, but this adds another dimension to our warrior's combat tasks. It affects our rules of engagement. Our soldiers must kill the enemy but must not harm noncombatants and must respect their property as well. The enemy knows this and frequently uses women and children as shields. They use mosques as safe havens for the same reason.

Adaptive Behaviors

The veteran combatants teach the fledgling warriors to distinguish between incoming and outgoing artillery and to hit the deck and not look out a door or window when they hear an explosion. New guys are cautioned not to bunch up and to avoid crowds. They show them how to drive down the middle of the road and what are the danger signs of an improvised explosive device or a vehicular-borne improvised explosive device. Structures built over the road are high risk for ambushes. Soldiers learn to keep nonmilitary vehicles at a distance by gesturing with weapons and sometimes throwing water bottles at them. They learn to be hypervigilant and to carry a weapon with them at all times. They are wary of people with bulky clothing, carrying a cell phone, and even women and children who approach them despite their orders to halt. A flash of light in the distance signals that someone is firing or about to fire at them.

Life-Saving, Reflex Reactions

Neurologically, the amygdala, a walnut-sized structure located in the temporal lobes of the brain, can evaluate an auditory stimulus in fifteen milliseconds and produce a startle reflex in which the warrior crouches and his pupils dilate, gut evacuates, heartbeat increases, blood pressure goes up, face grimaces and he prepares to run or fight. This adrenaline rush can cause a warrior to sweat in subzero temperatures and to freeze when it is hot as an oven outside. This is the adrenaline "high" that some soldiers miss. Combat soldiers must be hypervigilant and ramped up with adrenaline and yet calm and relaxed to be able to perform and shoot their weapons accurately. This is not a natural reaction but one that must be learned. Martial artists and boxers know that muscle tension inhibits the speed and power of their movements and yet they must be hyperalert and acutely aware of their surroundings and their opponent. They train and learn to develop upper-body relaxation while being fully aware and alert. (If you find yourself in a physical confrontation with another and your opponent takes a deep breath and relaxes, you know you are probably in big trouble.) Warriors need to keep their breathing slowed and their muscles relaxed while staying hyperalert. Hypervigilance often persists after returning home and is seen as a symptom of PTSD. Lack of emotion and detachment are also symptoms of PTSD and are carryovers from the combat environment.

The memory of the stimulus that produces the startle reaction is stored in the amygdala immediately, and the startle reaction can be evoked by anything closely resembling the trigger from then on. It is very specific and, for example, may be evoked by the sound of enemy bullets whizzing by but not by the louder explosions of friendly forces weapons. This reaction appears strange and out of place when evoked in a civilian environment.

Behaviors Unique to the Combat Zone

Some warriors develop the habit of urinating in a bottle in the morning rather than trudging to the latrine in the cold of Afghanistan or the heat of Iraq. They learn not to bunch up or congregate as a group, which provides an inviting target to insurgents. They go without sleep for long stretches of time and, when they do sleep, they do so with one eye open and a weapon close at hand. They become accustomed to the heat and the dust.

In the base camp soldiers follow the same routine nearly every day. They see the same people, eat the same food, follow the same schedule, and talk about the same topics. A good part of any tour involves coping with boredom. In Vietnam we took off our fatigues after dinner and wore our skivvies so we would know we were off duty. Guys would talk in detail for days about a lizard or a doughnut dolly they spotted. The day I arrived in the division a doctor, wearing only a towel and carrying a bar of soap, was walking to the outdoor shower a few feet away from where a group of physicians were sitting in their lawn chairs dressed in flip-flops and underwear shorts. One of the docs said to the fellow, "Where are you going?" The fellow in the towel said, "Going to the shower." Another doc asked, "Going to the shower?" "Yes," the fellow replied, "I'm going to the shower." Another doc said, "Let me know how the water is." "OK," the fellow with the towel replied. Later, as the fellow left the shower drying off, a doc asked, "How was the water?" "Wet," the soldier answered. This was met with laughter and then a long, detailed exchange about the temperature of the water. As a new guy I wondered what sort of doctors these were. I'd never heard such a dumb, detailed discussion about the obvious. A few months later I was sitting in a lawn chair with the other doctors drinking beer and a fellow in a towel was heading for the shower and I caught myself asking, "Going to the shower?"

Perceived Control Reduces Stress

Combat stress is correlated with the amount of control the individual feels he has over his situation. In a laboratory, rats were put on wire grids and were shocked periodically. If the rat was given a lever to push that would stop the shocks, the rat would stay at the lever, continually pushing it, and would not develop the physiological signs of stress. If the same rat was shocked randomly whether he pushed the lever or not, he would develop the stigmata of stress. In World War II it was observed that pilots, who had some control, developed less stress than turret gunners, who had no control over the aircraft. Fighter pilots, who seemingly had more control over their destinies, experienced less stress than bomber crews. Another study in World War II was conducted on the thousands of men who were initially screened out at induction centers with the diagnosis of "neuroses." So many men were being eliminated that there was concern that we would be unable to muster sufficient troops. Orders came down from the surgeon general to require these men to serve. A follow-up study was done to determine how these "neurotics" functioned in combat. To everyone's surprise it was discovered they performed better than soldiers who were felt to be "normal" psychologically. The theory was that in combat these men knew the source of their anxiety (the enemy who was shooting at them) and were able to do something about their fears (shoot back). This situation was more tolerable than walking around with free-floating anxiety and being unable to do anything about it. We observed more stress among engineers and MP crossing guards in Vietnam because when they were fired upon, they had less opportunity to return fire and felt less control.

Frustration and Anger

Warriors become short-tempered. The adverse climatic conditions (it was pretty hot in Vietnam, and the temperatures in Iraq exceed 130 degrees during the summer), fears of death and injury, primitive living conditions, long hours of boredom, loneliness, sexual tension, having to be constantly vigilant, and poor sleep all contribute to the soldier's irritability and smoldering anger. Soldiers are irritated with troops stationed behind them who have safer and more comfortable assignments. Soldiers who are on patrol outside of the wire surrounding the base camp tend to be irritated with those within. There is universal irritation toward the rear echelon mother-fucks, also known as the "beer in the rear" support troops.

Dependence on Comrades

In the field warriors learn to function as a unit. If they develop their skills as a coordinated group, it is more likely that they will perform optimally and survive in combat. If they fail to make their decisions based on the best interest of the group, it is likely that neither they nor their group will make it. The supremacy of the group over the needs of the individual is intensified in the combat area. Men sacrifice themselves for their comrades. The greatest support sustaining them in combat is the bond with their fellow soldiers. It is also the motivation that keeps them in the battle area when their primal survival urges tell them to leave. Men on sick leave in the hospital will volunteer to return to their units to help their buddies. Men will turn down opportunities to be evacuated out of loyalty to their units and their comrades in arms. Warriors have been trained to kill the enemy but only when ordered to do so and according to strict rules of engagement. This may cause conflicts for the warrior who has to make instantaneous decisions that may result in the death of women or children who may be carrying explosives. Failure to act may result in the death of the warrior or his comrades in arms.

Control and Preoccupation with Detail

Men who are the tip of the sword and outside of the wire are acutely aware that small details can mean the difference between life and death. Loose shoestrings, the snap of a twig, or the sound of loose gravel, a dirty weapon, or the clinking of two dog tags—any small error can lead to disaster not only for the individual but also for the entire unit. Combat units train constantly to minimize lost time and confusion in battle. For example, artillery units keep their equipment in the same locations so that any new man in the unit could, in the dark, locate wrenches, shells, or any standard piece of equipment immediately. Compulsive attention to detail is part of the warrior's training and is vital to his and his unit's survival in the combat zone.

Excitement and Adrenaline Highs

Warriors are doing what they have been trained to do. The experience of war is unique. There is horror and trauma, but there is also excitement and adventure. There is an intense closeness with comrades that is impossible to duplicate. I've seen a number of veterans who found it difficult to adjust back to civilian life and who re-upped to return to the peak experiences and close relationships they had in the combat zone.

Maintaining the Connection with Home

Communicate with your spouse and family at home. Write letters daily and number them. Try to fill them out with the details of your day but also try to avoid causing undue alarm. Try to be upbeat and positive in your letters and messages. Think about what the kids might be interested in seeing and hearing and describe events they might want to hear. For example, a dog that is a mascot, kids you've seen, and what they are doing. Be sure to tell your wife how much you appreciate the extra burdens she is shouldering at home and tell her and the kids how much you love and miss them. My girls were too young to read when I was in Vietnam, and so I drew cartoon figures and tried to put together pictures and letters so they would be able to figure them out themselves (i.e., "R U OK?" and then a picture of an eye accompanied by "M OK 2"). They had fun "reading" letters from Dad.

Send digital recordings and coordinate them with pictures you e-mail. You can narrate your slide/videotape show. You can record interviews with other guys in your unit and have them talk about the day's events (tell them to clean up the language for the family). Sing "Happy Birthday" to those at home to hear on their special days.

Warriors need to support their wives and families at home. Soldiers should recognize the heavy load they are carrying and thank their waiting spouses for all they are dealing with at home. They should reassure them that they miss them and love them. Send her a mushy romantic card. Send little gifts to her and to the kids. Make arrangements for one of her friends to take her out to dinner or to a movie as a surprise from you. Send her flowers.

Military Wife (or Husband) to Waiting Wife (or Husband)

Spouses frequently go through an initial stage of shock and disorientation when their soldier is deployed. Many say they spend the first few days crying and in shock as the reality of their spouse's departure sinks in. This is followed by a period of anger, frustration, and

IV: Deployment

depression. They may withdraw socially and find it difficult to push themselves to carry out their new responsibilities and expanded routine. One waiting wife suggested that wives should spend no longer than two hours in their pajamas and no more than a day in the house. This is where membership in a waiting wives group and having an experienced spouse mentor will help. The veteran will encourage the novice to get going and to get involved with others. Waiting wives (and waiting husbands) find they will be taking on responsibilities that are new to them.

The experienced wife will encourage the waiting wife to get going and establish a schedule for herself and her children. Soldiers are with their buddies and can focus on their jobs while families wait at home and wonder what is going on. Soldiers are surrounded by buddies who are in the same boat. Families at home are frequently in civilian surroundings where no one understands their situation. Schools may not understand the children's reactions. People may make comments about the war that are upsetting. News programs may show events that worry those waiting at home. Civilians have no understanding of how difficult life has become for the waiting families.

It is normal for waiting wives to experience a good deal of anger and frustration. Hillary Martin, author of *Solo-Ops: A Survival Guide for Military Wives*, says she wishes there was an 800 number you could call and yell at the military. She mentions a waiting wife who iron-transferred a picture of bin Laden to a pillow and then beat and screamed at it.

Shortly after the initial shock, numbness, sadness, and anger there may be a positive change as the waiting wife begins to look at the positives. There will be less mess to clean up. There will be less laundry to do. She will decide the schedule at home and be in control of the decision making. The emotionally draining predeployment wait for his departure is now over.

It is better if the waiting spouse and family can focus on their routines and jobs at home. A routine schedule provides security for everyone. Devise not only a daily list of chores and activities but also a meal plan that everyone can anticipate. For example, Monday a Crock-Pot or casserole meal; Tuesday, oriental; Wednesday, soup; Thursday, pasta; Friday, homemade pizza; Saturday steak; and Sunday, breakfast, church, followed by a full Sunday dinner. Knowing what to expect for a nice home-cooked meal provides security and comfort for the children. Have a nightly routine and include the missing parent in the ritual. Let them know that Daddy (or Mommy) is thinking about us back at home.

Make sure that you and your extended family give the kids plenty of hugs and kisses. Tell them that some of them are from the warrior.

For children who are in school, plan a time for homework and a time for you to review their work with them. Read to the children before bed on a regular basis.

Plan predictable, fun activities for the family. Watch a football game on Sunday. Have homemade pizza and a movie on Friday nights. Watch favorite television shows together with popcorn. Go for a walk or bicycle ride together.

Schedule chores for the children. Giving them regular duties and responsibilities will permit them to help you with the burden of maintaining the household during deployment. It gives them an opportunity to earn some spending money as well. Don't be surprised if the children test you to see if you hold to the new schedule. By keeping to your routine, you will give them security and the knowledge that you will be setting a predictable structure for them at home.

Take care of your appearance and your health. People who are depressed and overwhelmed with demands frequently neglect themselves, which only makes them feel worse and drains them further. Fixing yourself up, eating healthy foods, exercising, getting regular checkups, and attending to medical and dental problems will help you be at your best as you take on the extra burdens of parenting and managing the day-to-day household duties. Read a good book, join a gym, go to dinner with another waiting wife, hang out with positive friends, or join a Bible group or a self-help group or both.

Waiting male spouses should take care of themselves as well. Men are usually resistant to the idea of going to the doctor or dentist when they don't have an acute problem. They can benefit from the support of other waiting males, support groups, and/or professional caregivers.

Organize your budget and stay with it. You will have more money from his or her deployment with family separation pay, tax exclusions, hostile fire/imminent danger pay, hazardous duty pay, per diem, etc. You can determine the amount at www.militarymoney.com or www.military.com/benefits/military-pay. It is important to stay within the budget and save for contingencies while he is away. Financial stress can cause problems. This is one source of stress you can avoid through planning and discipline.

Try to limit your exposure to the news. Typically the news stresses the negative and the sensational from the combat zones. The Greeks in 500 BC had their melancholic patients watch comedies and listen to upbeat music. It is still good advice today. Try to read and watch upbeat and humorous material.

Get out and socialize with couples who have good marriages. Too often, deployed married couples get involved in extramarital affairs, and this leads to divorce in most cases. Surround yourself with people who are faithful to their warriors, and resist any temptation to stray yourself.

The same advice applies to the male spouse who looks after the kids at home with the additional admonishment that he recognizes that, as a male, he is going to resist the suggestion that he develop a support system for himself and the children. Also, he will have more difficulty recognizing and expressing his feelings.

Communication with the Warrior

One possible advantage to our slow communication in Vietnam was that it made it easier for us to detach from "the world" back home and focus on our day-to-day tasks in Vietnam. We didn't really think seriously about going home until we became short and, when we did, we then became fearful for our safety and reluctant to put ourselves at any risk. I don't know if the warriors in OIF or OEF were more anxious than we were as a result of having better connection with home. I do know of a Special Forces sergeant in Afghanistan whose dad had been a member of Delta in Vietnam. The sergeant called his father during a firefight and let him hear the gunshots and the conversations of his unit members while the battle was waging. This would be contraindicated in most situations, but this fellow's dad said he enjoyed hearing the action.

One point to keep in mind, although it is unlikely that your warrior will express this directly, is that soldiers are always angry with those behind them who have safer, more comfortable assignments (the rear echelon mother-fucks, or REMFs). This extends to civilians at home. He or she is likely to be irritable. He (or she) is proud of his family for handling the extra burdens at home and realizes you don't have it easy. However, he or she is living in an adverse climate in primitive surroundings with a large group of people trying to kill him or her. As a result, the warrior may have little patience for what seems to be petty complaints of the people back home. Should you, in all innocence, mention someone being upset by a minor inconvenience at home, you might anticipate that your warrior will feel and possibly react with some anger. (See the quote by George Hart at the beginning of this book.) Include your warrior in all decisions and changes that affect the family but realize it is unrealistic to think he or she can actually make decisions for home while being deployed. Try to make decisions you can both agree on. It is a good idea to be open and honest with your feelings, but don't put your warrior on the defensive. To do this, use "I feel" statements. You are always correct when you talk about your feelings, and you aren't saying that he or she made you feel that way—it is just sharing how you do feel. Don't take anger about separation and the extra demands you are dealing with out on your spouse. Let him or her know you appreciate how much they did when they were home, and how much you miss them and love them. Let your spouse know you will be a rock at home and not to worry about anything but getting back safely to you and the family.

Tell the children that you are going to maintain regular communication with your warrior and get them involved in writing, drawing pictures, and making cassette recordings and videos to send. Talk about the warrior daily with the kids. Get their ideas for funny letters and cards. Put the recorder on the dinner table and record the conversations. Record the sounds of the home (dog barking, birds chirping, and kids laughing) and talk about what you are doing. Bring the deployed warrior into the conversation with the kids whenever possible.

Set up a timeline poster or a basket of Hershey's kisses, or a paper chain numbered with the days of deployment, or something that the children can see daily as a concrete indicator of the time until the warrior returns. Some waiting spouses feel that a calendar or other indicator of the entire tour is too overwhelming and they pick twenty-five significant occasions over the year to use as markers (birthdays, holidays, etc.) and cross them out as they go by. If the child asks about dying, talk about it. Show the child on the calendar when your warrior will return and say that in the meantime, you will be thinking of and communicating with the deployed loved one. There is Buddy CJ, a CD-ROM that has games with a bear in a red T-shirt who talks about being upset that his parent was going on leave. The bear says things like, "Now I don't know what to think. I'm really sad."

Letters

Write daily and number the letters. Snail mail takes a long time, and it is easy for letters to get out of sequence and thereby become confusing. You each have a tape recorder and you can record cassettes for one another, and you may want to coordinate them with pictures you send by e-mail. Send local newspaper articles, jokes, pictures of your family, city, and state, and jokes you hear or read. Send a copy of the family schedule and chores and tell the soldier how important the routine has become for the children. Remind him that it will be important to continue the schedule for a while after he returns to give the children as sense of security and sameness as you try to develop a new family dynamic with Dad back in the picture. Send cartoons from magazines. Send jokes you hear. Take pictures of what you and the kids are doing all day, and send them in a letter. Send the kids' schoolwork. Have the kids draw pictures to send. I decorated my hootch in Vietnam with the kids' pictures, and it seemed more warm and homey. Send a digital recording of your day to accompany the pictures. Write down your sexual fantasies and use code words if you are afraid of someone else seeing what you are writing. Pick a day of the week to send erotic thoughts.

Postcards

Keep a stack of stamped, addressed postcards so the kids can write and mail one whenever they are in the mood to do so. Put one of these cards in your Christmas cards so that your friends and family can send a postcard to the warrior.

IV: Deployment

Digital Recordings and Videos

Record daily events at home (for example, dinner conversation with the family) and pretend your warrior is there with you. Keep him up-to-date with daily happenings. Let your soldier known you are all thinking of him, praying for his safety, and that you love him.

If he doesn't have access to some favorite TV shows or sports events, tape the shows for the warrior to watch overseas. Let the kids record their own messages.

Phone Calls

It is easy to forget what you wanted to discuss when you hear your warrior's voice. Keep some notes of events and things you want to say during your infrequent, brief calls. Carry a cell phone with you so he or she can always reach you whenever he or she calls. The reverse will not be true—the warrior will not be available when you want to talk. This is frustrating but just the reality of the situation. The warrior is probably going to call when you don't want to be interrupted. You may have just gotten into a good movie on the television or you might be enjoying a nice shower. It is normal to not feel like talking to your soldier at times. Remember that this reluctance is normal and nothing to feel guilty about or to cause concern about your relationship. If you don't want to be the first to hang up, count to three and hang up together. Record conversations so you can hear them again later and so the kids can hear their parent's voice.

E-mails

Remember that others may have access to the messages you send by computer. Try to keep messages brief and upbeat. Don't try to discuss emotional issues or get into arguments by e-mail. Let the kids get on the computer to e-mail the warrior as well. If you have private access to email you can flash each other on your webcam.

Care Packages

You can get more ideas from your soldier and also from reading lists of suggestions on the Internet, but here are some ideas of things to send. Have the kids help you prepare care packages for him or her. You might include some books the kids like so that he could read them to them on cassette tapes. Other items include books, board games, card games, comic books, electronic games, magazines, gossip newspapers, puzzles, footballs, Nerf balls, soccer balls, aspirin, Band-Aids, antacids, ChapStick, cough drops, dental floss, disposable razors, hairbrush, comb, Kleenex, mouthwash, Neosporin, Q-tips, soap, shampoo, Theraflu, toothbrushes, toothpaste, toilet paper, and wet wipes. Send homemade sweets (no chocolate), cookies, and fudge. Freeze cookies in a freezer bag and vacuum the air out of the bag. Updated photos, batteries, can opener, envelopes, gloves, gum, journal (to write in), pens, plastic utensils, stationery, hard candy, granola bars, beef jerky, beef sausage, canned meat, canned cheese, canned chips, canned salsa and dips, canned chicken, canned tuna, crackers, dried fruits, Hickory Farm treats, nuts, pretzels, individual packaged drinks (Kool-Aid, Country Time lemonade), clip-on flashlights, magazines, battery-powered socks if it's cold, battery-powered handheld fan if it is hot, MP3 player, iPod, cell phone with SIM card, Game Boy, DS, or PSP, and war games like *Soldiers of Anarchy* or *H.A.L.O.* Foot aids are also welcomed, which reminds me of a story about Vietnam. A battalion surgeon in Nam was being replaced by a doctor from the States. His company commander asked, "How's your turtle, Doc?" "He seems fine," answered the doc, "but he's a pediatrician, and I'm not sure how that will work." "Should work out fine, Doc," answered the CO. "We can use a good foot doctor around here." Dr. Scholl's gel insoles, fungus spray, foot powder, foot deodorant, and/or a foot massager are all helpful.

IV: Deployment

Pack a birthday cake and send it so it arrives on your warrior's birthday. Include a cassette of the kids and you singing "Happy Birthday." Send a pillow with your picture on it and tell him or her to hug it and think of you.

We've discussed some of the activities that will help prepare the soldier and the folks at home for the time apart during deployment. We noted some of the ways families have communicated and maintained their relationships while apart. The changes from soldier to warrior and from military dependent to single parent are described. Reversing many of these changes will be part of the postdeployment readjustment to civilian life. In the next chapter we'll discuss the period of deployment itself.

Section IV: Deployment

Chapter Four: Short—Pre-Entry—Anticipation of Homecoming

You've made it through the main part of the deployment, and both the warrior and the spouse and family at home have adjusted to the lengthy separation. Now you are approaching the warrior's return. He or she is "short," and you are both excited at the prospect of being together again.

This is an important period for both the warrior and the loved ones at home. Unrealistic expectations about it can lead to disappointment and frustration if they are not recognized and dampened in advance. In my forty years of private psychiatric practice, I've had an opportunity to work with many married couples. The peak time for stress in a marriage is in the early evening. These days many couples are both working, but for this example let us assume that the man is the breadwinner and the woman is a stay-at-home wife and mother. The man returns from work. He is tired and stressed from his day at the office. He is looking forward to returning to the peace and quiet of his home, to take his shoes off, to have a beer, turn on the television, and to be nurtured by his loving wife. The wife has been home with the children and is looking forward to her husband coming home, having an adult conversation, and sharing some of the demands she's been meeting all day. She anticipates his return to the house, relieving her of some of her burdens, and cuddling and nurturing her. What actually occurs is that two emotionally drained adults come together expecting the other one to meet his or her dependency needs, and they become frustrated and angry when they both feel deprived. It is easy to see how a greatly magnified version of the same frustration and anger may arise when a warrior, who has been dreaming and idealizing his return home for a year, gets together with his wife and children who have been similarly anticipating that their frustrations will be satisfied by Dad when he gets home. At the least, both the warrior and family will feel disappointed by the experience. At the most, there may be an emotional explosion of rage and withdrawal from one another.

Short

The warrior begins to count down the days on his or her short-timer's calendar. In Vietnam these were cartoons of naked women covered with numbers that the soldier colored in until he reached the final number. He yelled "short" when he awakened each morning, and he told his buddies things such as he didn't have time for a whole beer, had three more wakeups and a duffle bag drag (going home in three days), "I'm so short I have to stand on a dime to see over a nickel," he could listen only to 45 rpm records, wasn't able to start a book—only time for magazines, had to have ripe bananas, etc. His buddies would respond with stories of guys who were killed as they were leaving country, or, if he was returning to a military post in the continental United States (CONUS), they would tell him how great it was going to be that he could go to the commissary and buy cheap razor blades and how he was going to enjoy shining his boots every day.

Psychologically, men began to believe they were going to make it home when they got short. Up until that time they focused on their job in Nam and didn't think seriously about "the world." Once the warrior felt he was going to actually return to his loved ones, he became concerned about his personal safety. Command recognized this phenomenon and took men out of the field their final month in country.

Soldiers are likely to idealize their return home and their reunion with their spouses and families. They imagine things will be the same as when they left and that the family dynamics will be the same as well.

When you are short, it is a good time to review how you have changed and to imagine how the folks at home have moved on as well. You've learned to focus on the day-to-day events and not plan long-term into the future. You've suppressed your feelings. In Vietnam we used to say "Ain't no big thang" to cover any event, no matter how horrendous. You have had a regular schedule you've become used to following. You've become hypervigilant. You may react quickly to "triggers" such as crowded conditions, sudden movement, foreign cars, bulky clothing, certain odors, loud noises, or bright flashing lights. You may not feel comfortable without a weapon. You've been living in primitive conditions and may, for example, piss in a pop bottle or outside on the ground in the morning rather than trudging out to the latrine. You've become closely attached to your buddies and may feel that they are the only people outside of your family who count and the only ones who can truly understand you. You may have gotten accustomed to a largely male environment and using foul language. You may have lost some close friends and dealt with this trauma by withdrawing from others. You may be irritated at REMFs and particularly civilians who haven't shared your hardships or danger and who seem to be preoccupied with petty concerns. You may feel a smoldering anger for no particular reason and may flare up over petty comments. Try to think of constructive ways to vent your anger and frustration when you get back. Exercise is one good way. Talking with veteran buddies and your spouse is another. Alcohol and drugs are not a good idea and may cause other problems.

Remember how you have changed and how you will need to readjust to civilian life. The atmosphere, climate, water, food, and living conditions you've been used to for the past year will now change abruptly. In addition to the jet lag associated with the long flight home, you have probably developed habits of less than normal sleep and, when you do sleep, find that you are easily awakened. Military commanders accept four hours of sleep with brief naps as normal in a combat area. You will carry these sleep disturbances home with you when you return. You've learned to shut down your emotions other than anger. Being withdrawn and unemotional is going to seem weird to people who are excited about seeing you and looking forward to your happiness at seeing them and being home again. The schedule you've been used to no longer exists. Peeing in a bottle, swearing, and packing a gun will make you stand out back in Middle America. You've become hypervigilant. You sit with your back to the wall and scan anyone who looks suspicious. You are obsessed with checking details and try to control things to prevent a fatal error.

Diving for the deck when you hear a car backfire or lying down in the front seat while driving when you see the bright reflection of the sun on a window is viewed as odd behavior at home. Some of the stimuli that trigger a protective reaction can be sounds and sights that ordinary civilians do not understand. Toyota, Nissan, and other Asian-made vehicles are common on today's battlefield, and a certain model or color of these cars can cause instant flashbacks. Newly returned veterans may drive rapidly down the middle of the road in the United States looking for IEDs. Some OIF veterans described having the urge to throw a water bottle at automobiles that approached them too closely stateside based on this habit overseas. I remember sitting in the right front seat of my jeep in

Saigon motioning with my .45 for vehicles to move away from us in areas where the traffic was congested. As Al Capone used to say, "A kind word with a gun in your hand will accomplish more than a kind word alone." You may have seen close friends injured or killed, and you may feel guilty that you made it while they didn't. You may have killed the enemy, and now you have a chance to think about it and to reflect on their humanness and your own guilt for taking a life. You may have memories of close friends who were killed or injured and feel guilty for having made it while they didn't. You'll probably still be struggling about the morality of your actions and will, no doubt, show some of the seemingly irrational behavior carried over from the combat zone.

In addition to the changes you've undergone through training and adjusting to the combat zone, you have changed as a result of the stress you've been under while deployed. For example, some of the dampening down of your feelings is due to your training and conscious effort to do so in order to be focused and alert during battle. Some, however, is automatic as your body responds to a surge in adrenaline that is the result of your exposure to stress. As you probably know, stress causes a release of steroids from the adrenal gland that produce a "flight or fight reaction" in the body. Your pupils dilate, your heart rate increases, you become hypervigilant, your rate of breathing increases, your gut evacuates, your muscles tense, and you are ready to fight or run. As a warrior you are trained to utilize this reaction to function under battle conditions. This reaction occurs not only in the heat of battle but also in the day-to-day life of the so-called support troops. They live under adverse conditions and with the constant threat of IEDs, car bombs, rockets, mortars, snipers, and individual suicide bombers. Veterans are sometimes of the opinion that just because they weren't kicking down doors and shooting people, they are immune to stress reactions, such as the later development of post-traumatic stress disorder or other post-deployment mental health difficulties. I can attest to the fact that in Vietnam we saw acute combat stress reactions among the 15 percent of the warriors who served in the field, but the majority of the mental health cases we evaluated and treated came from the 85 percent of the men who were designated as support troops. It has now been recognized that PTSD can result from exposure to an acute traumatic event or, more commonly, from the cumulative effect of a series of traumatic stressors. Male or female soldiers who were abused in childhood or experienced sexual trauma are more vulnerable to developing PTSD from combat.

It is good to think in advance of your homecoming how you have changed since you were deployed and how these behaviors might seem out of place in the civilian environment. While you are at it, imagine how much your family has changed while you have been gone. Imagine what their fantasies are about your return. Your wife (or husband) has been carrying a double load all year. (I will refer to the waiting spouse as a female, but the same applies to the waiting male spouse.) She is looking forward to your stepping in and taking over some of the demands of the children and the household. She's been sending you care packages and trying to boost your morale while worrying about your safety. She is looking forward to having you home safe and sound to give her some of the nurturing care she's been missing. She wants to hear how much you appreciate all she did while you were gone and to see how much you loved and missed her while you were apart from one another.

Your spouse has been making all of the decisions. She may have included you in a few, but essentially she has been the boss. She may want to turn over some of the demands she's been meeting while you were away, but she may not be as quick to give up some of the authority she's taken on. The kids are used to looking to Mom for answers, and they will continue to do so when you return. They may have turned to substitute father figures during your absence. Don't be upset if they continue to do so until they get used to your presence in the family. Your wife will try to include you or tell them to "Ask your daddy," but they are used to her being the boss. You may initially feel as though you are not needed by the family and pull back (which is what you are inclined to do anyway). Withdrawal from the family would be the wrong thing to do. Hang in there and you will again find your place with them. It won't be the same role it was before you left, but they want Dad there with them and you will find you are needed in the long run. Your wife and kids have a routine that they've been hanging on to for security while you've been absent from the home. They will be reluctant to let go of their security blanket or to change it initially. Go with the flow and try to fit into what they've been accustomed to doing while you were away. Find out what their schedule has been and follow it. If they have homemade pizza and movies on Friday, jump in and join them. You may find that you are bored with the home environment. You may find that the noise and demands of the children irritate and frustrate you. Resist your temptation to go out with your buddies for a beer and stay with the family for the first few weeks.

You may be focused on the big honeymoon with your spouse, which is great, but don't forget the kids and their excitement about being with you as well. If you and Mom exclude them, it will make them feel that they aren't as important to you. Make sure you spend time with them and show them you love them and missed them.

These are important things to consider before you actually get together.

The Family's Expectations of Homecoming

Major John Morris uses a canoe as a metaphor when speaking to participants of a Family Integration Academy in Brooklyn Park, Minnesota. He describes how the leaving and returning of a deployed service member rocks a family the same way getting in and out of a canoe destabilizes it. Everyone in the family must work to balance the canoe.

(VFW June/July 2007. *The Road Home,* by Shannon Hanson. Page 15.)

The media pictures men in battle throughout the year and then give them adulation and thanks when they return. In contrast, the media may have showed a few wives waving good-bye to the troops at the airport and then embracing them when they returned. There are no news stories about the double burdens they took on during the soldier's year of absence. Soldiers are surrounded by their buddies, who are in the same situation and are supportive. The waiting wife may be isolated in a civilian environment surrounded by people who have no empathy for her situation. She likely kept her frustrations and loneliness to herself, not wanting to upset her warrior, who was risking his life in primitive surroundings in service to his country. She idealized his return and hoped that he would nurture her and relieve her of some of the emotional and physical demands she had been under for their time of separation. It is important for the spouse and the children to think about the upcoming reunion in advance. First they need to think about how much they have changed. Dad used to be a major authority figure and decision maker in the house. For the past year Mom has been the boss and making the decisions at home. The family has been following a regular schedule. Now you will have Dad back home, and he has been on his own schedule overseas. He may have forgotten that you go biking or for a walk on Wednesdays or that you like to have homemade pizza and movies on Fridays. While deployed he has been living under daily stress of a primitive, dangerous, largely male environment for a year. He has seen things he didn't describe to you because he didn't want to upset you and because he doubted that you could really know what he was saying. He may have done things that make him feel sad and guilty. He may feel guilty that his friends died or were injured and he was OK. He has had to learn behaviors to survive in a hostile environment. He will be in that environment up until a few hours before he arrives home. One veteran from Afghanistan told me he was shooting people within fifty meters less than twenty-four hours before he returned to the United States. This didn't give him very long to shed his combat habits or to adjust to the idea of a civilian environment. The same veteran went to work a short time after his return and had a Middle Eastern boss. He quit his job for fear he might lose control and injure his supervisor.

The spouse may be thinking that everything is going to be wonderful with her warrior back in the house. She may imagine that she will have a perfect honeymoon and then he will step in and relieve her of many of the burdens she's assumed during his absence. He will share the parenting of the children and will nurture and love her. Remember, he is likely thinking along the same lines. He may be looking forward to being home and being nurtured and cared for with none of the stress and demands he has been under for the past year. Warriors learn to suppress their feelings. Expecting him to be joyous at being home and seeing her and the children may seem like a demand to him. He may feel left out when the children turn to Mom and the family is following a schedule that is unfamiliar to him. The petty gripes that civilians have may be irritating to him after living in primitive conditions and seeing his comrades injured and killed. Questions about his year overseas may bring back upsetting memories to him. He will not describe traumatic events to protect his spouse and because he doesn't think she could really know what his experiences were like. He may be trying to avoid being hyperalert and to watch his language and behavior, which may also cause him to appear quiet and inhibited.

Patience is the watchword for both the returning warrior and the family. The behaviors of a year's duration cannot be altered at once.

It will take time for the warrior to let go of his habits and to adjust to civilian life again. It will take time for the family to adjust to his presence and to learn to depend on him again as a father and husband. Nevertheless, being aware in advance of the changes in both the warrior and the family that have taken place over the past year and of the unrealistic expectations that both have had will enable each to be more objective about their upcoming reunion. You've each been going your own way for a year. Give each other lots of time to adjust.

This chapter discussed the warrior's patterns of behavior in the combat zone and how the family coped with his or her absence from the home. Both the soldier and the family have had unrealistic fantasies about this reunion. Now it is time for the homecoming everyone has been dreaming of for the past year. It is a time of relief, joy, and affection. It is also wise to be realistic and lower everyone's expectations. The family and the warrior have changed and will now have to adjust and change once more. It is a time to exercise patience and tolerance for one another's problems adjusting.

Preparing for the Reunion

It would be better if both the warrior and the family could try to lower their expectations for the reunion. Think about the changes you all have made during your time apart. The expectation that everyone and everything will be the same as they were prior to deployment is not realistic. Everyone and everything will be different, but that isn't necessarily bad—in many cases it is good. Recognize that both the warrior and the family are hoping to be nurtured and relieved of demands and that these expectations are not realistic. It would be helpful for the warrior and the family to recognize the burdens each has borne during deployment and to thank each other for their service and their sacrifices over the past year.

The priest in Hemmingway's *For Whom the Bell Tolls* defines love as "To want to do things for." Jean-Paul Sartre said, "There is no love apart from the deeds of love." It is time to "walk the walk" and show your spouse through little acts of kindness and affection that you love him or her. Make an effort to nurture and coddle each other, and try to avoid making too many demands of one another. Be patient with each other. You've been apart for a long time and it will take a long time to readjust to each other again. Remember you love each other and you both want this relationship to be the best.

Section V: Postdeployment

Chapter Five: Honeymoon

From the Soldier's Perspective

You've been thinking and dreaming of the return home for the duration of your deployment. Your planeload of buddies and you cheer as you lift off the ground and again when you touch down back in the States. Your family is waiting for you with excitement and expectation. You know you should be euphoric, but strangely you find yourself feeling distant and out of place at home. You may have to fake the reaction of joy and excitement you know your family is expecting from you, but if you do, you feel like a hypocrite and you wonder why you have to act rather than just experience the joy of the moment.

This is a normal experience. A few hours ago you were in a hostile environment where you've spent the past year. Now you are going back through the looking glass and leaving the parallel existence of the combat zone. You are going to have to make the transition from a military to a civilian mind-set, and this won't be accomplished over night. Intellectually you may know you are back home and how you are supposed to react, but it takes time for your emotions to adapt to the change. Remember that your family is going through a similar adjustment. Intellectually they know they should be thrilled to have you back home with them, but emotionally it probably feels strange to be with you again. You need to be patient with your loved ones as they adjust to your return.

When we returned from Vietnam we were sometimes met with anger from civilians, sometimes taunted, and frequently ignored. One veteran told me two civilians told him he stunk. In Vietnam the locals washed our clothing in a polluted river and our feces was burned daily, which caused the air to have a peculiar odor. The combination of body odor from our sweat, the polluted water in which we bathed, plus contaminants in the water and air in our clothing caused us to stink. As one vet said, "We were beyond 'odor'—we went to 'o dear.'" We grew accustomed to the smells and were surprised when civilians on R&R or home told us we reeked.

It is helpful if you can share positive experiences about your deployment and your mission to help your family feel that the sacrifices and stresses they've gone through were meaningful and served a good purpose. It is useful for you to reflect on this as well. Your fellow countrymen are proud of you and grateful for your service, and it is not self-serving for you to feel good about what you've done and accomplished for your country. Don't forget to compliment your spouse on all she or he has done and accomplished while you've been away. You are the returning hero, but she or he is the unrecognized hero. Your spouse needs to hear that her worries and sacrifices are recognized and important.

You've learned to suppress your feelings, and you probably want to withdraw from the emotional demands you feel at home. Remember your family has been waiting all year for this day and looking forward to a joyful reunion. They want to see that you are happy to see them and glad to be home. The kids may be somewhat hesitant about greeting you and will no doubt turn to their mom (or dad) and to the substitute parental figures they've depended on while you were away. Be patient with them and let them get used to your presence. You may be eager to get to the honeymoon with your mate, but you want to pay attention to the kids and let them know you love them and missed them for the past year.

Your family has developed a routine to help them survive without you. It has worked for them. Don't try to alter what they've been accustomed to over the past year. Don't try to share your deployment stories initially. After everyone is used to having you back you can work in some of the war stories. You may be reluctant to do this, but they are curious about your experiences during your time apart from them. Tell them about your life while you were gone, but leave out material you think might gross them out. Take an interest in the family's activities and their growth while you were gone. Don't jump in and try to discipline the kids. Your spouse has been the disciplinarian. You can back your mate up, but don't try to take over. If you disagree about some aspect of their discipline, talk to your spouse in private about it and come to an agreement.

Laurie B. Slone, PhD, and Matthew J. Friedman, MD, PhD, in their book *After the War Zone: A Practical Guide for Returning Troops and Their Families*, note that *"After long flights, handshakes of thanks, and hugs and kisses, all the troops really want for the first few months when they come home is beer, sex, and pizza."* A note on the sex: To paraphrase Jeff Foxworthy, women are like diesel engines. It takes quite a while to get them warmed up, but then they can run a long time. Men are more like bottle rockets.

You may expect extra attention and nurturing when you return home. Remember that your spouse and children are expecting the same from you. This is a time to relax and get to know each other once more. It isn't a time to solve problems.

After the initial honeymoon, you and your spouse will need to discuss how the events of the past year have changed each of you.

You've both matured and gained confidence in yourselves. Some deployed soldiers feel they've aged as a result of their combat experience. Your observational skills may have improved. You've both achieved a degree of independence during the past year. Your roles in the family probably have to be redefined and readjusted. Your relationship with one another has changed, but this does not need to be a negative. The important thing is to listen to one another and remember that you love and want the best for each other. Be patient. You've both gone through a year's worth of changes, and it will take time to share what has happened and to understand one another.

Try to focus on the good. Just as the easier and safer assignment of the REMFs overseas may have irritated you, the civilians at home who have forgotten about the war and who seem preoccupied with petty concerns may be irritating as well. Returning veterans frequently look at civilians and think, "Where were you when I was away from my family, getting shot at, and putting up with the crummy living conditions overseas?" This sort of thinking leads the veteran to care less about the opinions of civilians at home. One former POW pretty much did what he wanted when he returned without regard to what anyone thought of his behavior. His favorite saying was "I'm not running a popularity contest." Instead of dwelling on resentment and bitterness toward civilians, think how your experiences have helped you mature and gain a perspective on life. You have been confronted with your own mortality, and as a result you are able to see what are the truly important things in life. You have been through a hardship tour and no longer take for granted the simple comforts of civilian life. You've been in danger and realize how important safety and security are at home. Absence from your loved ones has helped you realize that their relationships and love are the most important things in life for you. The bonds you formed with your comrades in arms have created lasting friendships as well.

We've described the typical homecoming of the average soldier as it will hopefully occur. Unfortunately things are not always so easy. One airborne unit had over forty cases of spousal abuse the first night the men arrived home. Some of the wives had been unfaithful, many were pregnant, and many had spent all of the money the returning veterans thought was in savings. Another unit reported that out of 146 returning soldiers, twenty wives had sold their houses, spent all of their money, gotten pregnant, and/or been bar hopping and unfaithful to their returning veterans. In 2002 the much-publicized killing of four wives by returning Special Forces soldiers occurred. I mention these extreme examples to illustrate that the return home can be extremely traumatic and explosive in a few cases. In most of these incidents, infidelity and financial stress appear to be the triggering events.

The Waiting Spouses' Perspective

You've been waiting for this day, but you probably feel a little anxious about the reunion. You want his homecoming to be perfect. It would probably be a good idea to lower your expectations for the event. Neither of you is the same as you were when he was first deployed. He will be a little quiet and distant. Typically returning veterans have problems communicating and being intimate. This is normal and something that time will usually heal. The warrior has had experiences that may be difficult to share and that you may never be able to really know even when he or she does describe the events to you. The warrior has to readjust to civilian surroundings. Some of his or her reserve is an effort to try to act appropriately, to watch his or her language, and to avoid using learned behaviors from the combat zone that are likely to surprise and shock the family at home. For example, the warrior may be easily startled when approached from behind, by sudden movements in his or her peripheral vision, light flashes, loud noises, Middle Eastern individuals, bulky clothing, trash on the side of the road, and/or people getting into his or her space. Be patient and let the veteran take the time to get used to everything again. Don't be surprised if the warrior is too exhausted from his or her flight and the demands of getting ready to leave country to react to your homecoming celebration.

You may be thinking that your warrior is going to take over the extra load you've been carrying and to provide you with the love, support, and nurturing you've been missing during his absence. If you think about this, he or she is probably hoping the same from you. You may both feel frustrated when your desire to lean on your partner is frustrated. You may feel a smoldering anger because of the demands you have both been under the past year and the feeling that your partner fails to recognize or to appreciate your burdens.

Karen M. Pavlicin, in her book *Surviving Deployment*, suggests that you and your warrior take time to grieve together over the loss of your time together, the experiences you each went through without the other, and the losses of friends who were killed. Look at the good things that came out of the year apart, such as the ways you each grew as individuals. Thank your spouse for his or her service to our country and for making the world safer for you and the family. Remember that you and your children have shared in the sacrifice for your country and deserve credit as well. Your separation from one another has reminded you how important your marriage and love for one another is. Your concern for his or her safety has reminded you of your own mortality and the brevity of life. This helps you reflect on what you feel are the true values in life.

When he or she is ready, let your warrior express any guilt about surviving when his or her comrades did not. Permit your spouse to talk about his or her feelings about taking the lives of the enemy if this is on his or her mind. You may want to share your feelings about losing the time together and the experiences you were unable to share with one another. Take it slow and be patient. Remember you love each other and, while you aren't the same as you were when you left one another, you've both matured and developed over the past year.

Posthoneymoon

After the joy of the reunion and honeymoon, problems may begin to surface. There may be differences of opinion about your routine at home. You may run into differences as to how to discipline the children, trust issues, suspiciousness, jealousy, money worries, and disagreements about household rules. Be patient. Talk calmly about your concerns and differences. It is understandable. You've been separated for an extended period, and it is going to take some time to reestablish the family dynamics again. Remember the core is you love each other and your relationship and family are important to all of you. Be patient with one another. You both had a demanding year, and you both are probably a little disappointed that you didn't receive all of the nurturing you were anticipating now that you are together again.

The children are likely to act up a little at this stage. Preschool children may have made something for the returning parent. They may be oppositional and avoid the returning parent who left them, or they may be clingy and seek constant attention. Children in elementary school may also be attention seeking or show temper tantrums. They may play one parent against the other to see if they are truly united again. Teenagers may be defiant and have problems at school or with their behavior. The service member should be patient and loving and not try to assert his or her authority initially. Support the parent who has been home doing double duty.

Posthoneymoon Advice for the Returning Warrior

- Be patient. This is a good but big adjustment for you. Expect chaos for a few days until you and your family settle down. Some Guard and Reserve units have a ninety-day leave before returning to their civilian jobs.

- Get some sleep. You are probably sleep deprived and you have jet lag from your flight home.

- Don't drink. There is a temptation to self-medicate with alcohol and to celebrate to the extreme. Your tolerance probably is much less than you remember it being. This can get you into difficulties.

- Don't drive. Road rage is common among returning veterans, who also may be in the habit of driving fast down the middle of the road to avoid IEDs.

- Don't try to change things.

- You've been dealing with life-and-death situations and living in a stressful environment. Naturally, civilian life and concerns will seem petty by comparison.

- Leave your weapons locked up. You are used to having a weapon in the combat zone. You don't need it at home, and having one can lead to serious problems and a risk for family members.

- Recognize and accept the changes that have occurred while you were away.

- Spend as much time at home as you can. You may want to check out your buddies or have beers at the VFW, but hold that until later. This is the time to reunite with the family. Even if the kids seem to ignore you and turn to your spouse, hang in there. They are making sure you are going to be around.

- Follow the routine they have used while you were gone. If Friday is pizza and a movie, join right in.

- Don't try to tell your spouse how to run the house more efficiently or make suggestions about finances.

- Let the spouse handle the discipline and support her (or him) when she (or he) does.

- You want to spend time with your wife, but don't exclude the children—they've been waiting to be with you, and they need you.

- Don't try to take over discipline of the children. Support your spouse.

- If your sex isn't what you dreamed it would be, talk about it together. Good sex is a by-product of a good, comfortable, relationship. If you love each other and can talk about it, you'll be fine.

- Decisions about the future career choices (for example, whether to remain in the military or not) and education need to be made and agreed upon with the spouse and the family.

Posthoneymoon Advice for the Waiting Spouse

- Be patient and don't push your warrior to jump back into his or her old role with the family.

- Anticipate changes in your spouse.

- He or she has been regimented for a year and may rebel against being told what to do. Be flexible.

- Remember he (or she) hasn't been getting restful sleep.

- There are lots of survival behaviors that are no longer needed but will take time to shed.

- You are proud of the way you handled everything on your own. Your spouse is too, but he or she may also feel a little hurt and worry that you and the kids may not need him or her. Reassure your spouse that you do.

- Recognize that you both were hoping to be "babied" and nurtured. Do a little pillow fluffing and butt coddling.

- Remember both of you need time together to get used to one another again and to drop some of the adaptive behaviors you've developed while you were apart. Don't push. Be patient.

- Don't expect your warrior to share his or her year's experiences or to be able to open up and tell you what is on his or her mind. If the warrior is a guy, remember, guys don't usually know how they feel, and if they should figure out what they are feeling, they are reluctant to express those feelings. Also, if you ask him what he is thinking and he says "nothing"—it is possible. This is often surprising to women, who are always thinking something—men's brains are frequently blank! One comedienne said that women use five thousand words a day while men use two thousand. They are silent at the end of the day because they've run out of words.

- When you do try your hand at problem solving together, give each other slack and listen to one another. Try to reach a mutual agreement.

- Talk about your conclusions and evaluate what you've accomplished together. Give each other some strokes for being such a great team.

Posthoneymoon Communication

Both of you may have feelings of anger and insecurity. You need to discuss and express these feelings. Talk about the expectations you had for the reunion. Discuss the good and the bad aspects of your current situation.

If you run into conflicts, identify what it is. Use "I feel" statements that are nonthreatening and nonaccusatory. Look for solutions together. What are the alternatives? Remember this is the person you love in life and who loves you. Avoid statements that are hurtful. If you do inadvertently say something that injures your partner, apologize immediately. Listen to your partner's comments knowing that they love you and what they say is in your best interest.

Helping the Children

Spend as much time as possible with the children after deployment, even if they withdraw, ignore you, and turn to your spouse. Just listen to them, pay attention to them, and tell them you love them. Help them get reacquainted with you.

Let them know that it is OK for them to express their feelings, including negative ones. You might discuss the normality of being angry with a parent who leaves for an extended period—even though you logically know it wasn't your parent's choice and he or she was doing a patriotic deed for the country. Make sure they don't feel excluded as you and your spouse spend time together. Visit their teachers and classrooms. Show interest in what they are and have been doing while you were away.

It is normal for children to show changes in eating and sleeping patterns, to be clingy, to have temper tantrums, to worry about safety, to show changes in academic performance, to have physical complaints, to withdraw, and to have a loss of interest in their usual activities.

Section VI: Normal Reactions to Abnormal Situations and Readjusting to Home

Eighty-five percent of veterans come home, utilize the programs and assistance provided by the military, and both they and their families make the adjustment. The number of mental and family problems increases with each deployment they go through. The media have emphasized the problems that have occurred among the minority of returning veterans and perhaps, in some cases, exaggerated the extent and severity of problems in the service of sensationalism. Much of the way we feel comes from our attitude toward our circumstances. It is important for your morale to maintain a positive outlook and not let yourself be negatively influenced by the news. As I was leaving my dermatologist's office, he said, "Stay out of the sun." "Why?" I asked. "Do I have something that would cause me to avoid the sun?" "No," he answered, "I say that to all of my patients—don't you psychiatrists have something you say to all of your patients?" I thought for a moment and then said, "Don't watch the news?" I mention this because veterans should stay upbeat and give themselves a pat on the back as trained professionals and for going through a stressful experience and extended separation from their loved ones and then readjusting to civilian life or stateside service. Families should also be complimented for coping at home and supporting their deployed warriors. You are strong people and you've faced a stressful experience and, in most cases, coped with it.

Not all families have a soldier who returns from deployment and gradually adapts to civilian life or a stateside assignment. Some warriors have a few weeks home to reconnect, which according to one veteran is just long enough to find out how far out of the loop he was. Then he has to start retraining, going to school, and probably relocating. All of these activities interfere with "coming home." Some don't make the adjustment, and these men and women suffer from more severe, long-lasting problems that will be discussed in the next chapter.

All returning soldiers are given the Post-Deployment Health Assessment (PDHA) or DD Form 2796. This provides a record of their self-reported symptoms at the time they returned to the continental United States (CONUS). The reported psychological problems are usually fairly low in this initial report because the soldiers are still in a military setting (they haven't encountered the stresses of adjustment to civilian life), they don't want to be delayed getting home, and they are still in shock after having just flown back from the combat area. A few weeks later they are given the Post-Deployment Health Reassessment (PDHRA), self-report Form DD2900, and interview. More difficulties are reported at this time. Typically, veterans underreport their symptoms and problems on both occasions because there remains a general concern that to be totally forthcoming would reflect badly on them and might endanger future promotions and security clearances. All veterans will have some changes due to their experiences while deployed. If you examine your own situation, you will observe that all spouses and families experience changes in themselves during the period of separation. Now that you are reunited, you will need to readjust to being together in a civilian milieu. Patience, love, and time will enable most warriors and families to make these readjustments. While the majority of veterans and families adjust without help, this does not mean that their adaptations could not have been

Section VI: Normal Reactions to Abnormal Situations and Readjusting to Home

made easier or that some of the problems they had could not have been lessened had they had some assistance. This chapter will focus on some of the common patterns and ideas for facilitating readjustment for the majority of warriors who will do so without seeking professional assistance. If problems persist, worsen, or are more than you seem to be able to handle, you may need professional assistance, which will be the subject of the next chapter.

The lengthy title of this chapter describes the conditioning during military training that enables the soldier to relinquish his inhibitions against killing and to subvert his individuality to that of the combat group. It refers as well to the normal adjustments a warrior makes to the stressful combat situation. Suppression of feelings, hypervigilance, focus on the mission, secrecy, controlled aggression, and attention to detail are all adaptive behaviors in a war zone. He developed and utilized these new behaviors to survive for a year while he was deployed. Within a short time the warrior has been flown home and now has to drop these behaviors and readjust to civilian life. Obviously this will take time. The behaviors the warrior exhibits are strange and out of place in the civilian environment but were normal where he or she has been for the past year. Males in particular tend to want to solve their own problems and tend to turn to compulsive behaviors in an effort to make themselves feel better. One of these is self-medication with drugs and/or alcohol. This should be avoided, as it tends to make everything worse and may result in an additional problem in itself. The answer is to utilize conditioning techniques to modify the warrior's learned actions into civilized, socially acceptable patterns of behavior.

Returning female warriors have all of the adjustments men have and more. They switch from the masculine warrior role to a feminine nurturing role when they return home. They now cook, clean, and care for the children. Men, on the other hand, essentially step into the same masculine role they had before deployment.

You now have greater awareness of the changes warriors experience in training and combat. You may not know that the peculiar behaviors warriors exhibit when they return are normal reactions to the abnormal experiences of war. Soldiers are more aware of the changes their families have undergone during their absences from home. In contrast to previous wars, particularly Vietnam, society is understanding and supportive of returning warriors and their families. Soldiers in the voluntary military, in general, are better trained, more motivated, and have a positive attitude toward their service. On the other hand, many drafted soldiers during the Vietnam era were educated and highly trained. (For example, among my social work psychology technicians in Nam I had a PhD psychologist who was a forward artillery observer, a "tunnel rat" who was a probation officer, a PhD in anthropology who was a conscientious objector, and several trained social workers.) In general, the families of our current soldiers share a positive outlook toward the military and the mission. All of these factors contribute to the current warrior's positive adjustment during the postdeployment stage. On the negative side, OIF and OEF warriors have been redeployed more with less recovery time between their hardship assignments than veterans of previous conflicts.

The military has developed programs to teach soldiers mental toughness. The army's program is called BATTLEMIND and was developed by Colonel Carl Castro, PhD, at Walter Reed Medical Center. Breaking down the components of the mnemonic, I will point out the trait that is useful in battle and the possible negative effect of this characteristic if continued in civilian life postdeployment.

BATTLE MIND

Buddies are the ones warriors depend on in combat. They have your back and they share your unique experience. At home the veteran may miss his close comrades, and he may want to hang out with them after his return home. He may feel they are the

Section VI: Normal Reactions to Abnormal Situations and Readjusting to Home

only ones who really understand him, and he may feel safe in their presence.

Accountability in battle is where everyone is responsible for their actions and the consequences of their behavior. This may become a problem postdeployment if the warrior becomes upset with anyone doing anything with his possessions or fails to take responsibility for him- or herself. The warrior may be overly strict and have a hard time letting things go.

Targeted Aggression and Tactical Awareness. These traits may help the warrior survive in a dangerous war zone, but they may carry over into inappropriate aggression, as well as keyed-up, hypervigilant, anxious behavior. The warrior may have a startle reaction when confronted with any of the triggers that remind him of combat (loud noises, flashes of light, people of ethnic groups who dress or look similar to the enemy, people getting too close to him, piles of garbage on the side of the road, bulky clothing, etc.).

Lethally Armed. It's appropriate to have a weapon in a war zone but inappropriate and dangerous at home. Many warriors do not feel safe without their loaded weapon being within reach.

Emotional Control. Expression of emotions is discouraged and mental toughness is encouraged at war. A warrior may appear emotionally detached and remote at home. Other times he or she may show outbursts of anger over seemingly minor situations.

Mission Security. Warriors talk about missions only on a need-to-know basis in combat area. At home, they may seem secretive.

Individual Responsibility is important in a war zone, but at home he may feel guilty for men who were injured or died, feeling that he was responsible in some way for their deaths or for not being able to protect them. He may also have survivor's guilt for having lived while some of his buddies didn't make it.

Nondefensive Driving. He may drive fast down the middle of the road. He may become angry and want to throw a water bottle at cars that come too close to his automobile.

As previously described, there is a similar BATTLEMIND mnemonic for spouses of deployed warriors. The important points are that the waiting wife has taken over the job of both parents and the household duties during the warrior's absence. It is important to plan ahead how the couple will divide up the responsibilities when the warrior returns. Control at home will have to be renegotiated. The warrior may think things will be as they were when he left. The spouse and family at home are well aware of the time, as they counted each day following deployment. The couple needs to be patient with one another and talk things out. Loyalty and commitment during deployment are important for both and for the stability of the relationship.

Resiliency Training

Army Chief of Staff General George W. Casey Jr. was looking for a reliable approach to prepare the army's 1.1 million soldiers for the adjustment from combat to civilian life. Comprehensive Soldier Fitness, which aims to develop each soldier's mental, physical, spiritual, social, and family health, was already in place. Under this general program the military utilized resiliency training that was originally created by Karen Reivich and Andrew Shatte at the University of Pennsylvania to help high school students do well under pressure and to adapt when confronted with adversity. The government invested $117 million to adapt their program to the army's unique requirements. Sergeants are going through resiliency instructor training so that they will be equipped to train the troops.

Section VI: Normal Reactions to Abnormal Situations and Readjusting to Home

This program has also been extended to training family members to deal with adversity and, specifically, the stress of their loved one's deployment. For example, a spouse might be asked to think of the worst thing that might happen to her deployed warrior (being killed in battle) and the best thing (winning a lot of money, promotion, etc.) and then helped to see that the likely reality was somewhere between the two. The stress of deployment was examined as a possible time for growth for both the warrior and the spouse in terms of increased independence, self-confidence, and the realization that both could be proud that they were sacrificing for the benefit of their country.

The idea of training military personnel in psychotherapy techniques to enable them to assist large numbers of personnel is not new. From 1930 to the early 1970s in the United States, psychiatry was dominated by psychoanalysis. To become a trained analyst in the United States in the 1940s, one had to complete college, medical school, internship, and psychiatric residency, and then complete analysis yourself and successfully analyze two patients under supervision. There was concern that there were far too few analysts to meet the needs of the millions of servicemen who required mental health attention. Carl Rogers developed an approach known as "Rogerian psychotherapy" in which therapists with minimal training would rephrase and reflect a patient's statements back to them.

Psychoanalysts at the time had a sick joke about this type of treatment:

A patient ran into a Rogerian therapist's office and said: "You've got to help me. I am terribly depressed."

Rogerian therapist (RT): "You feel a need for professional assistance because you are so despondent."

Patient: "Yes, that is correct. In fact, I am thinking of suicide."

RT: "You are so depressed that you feel the only way you can gain some control over your pain would be to take your own life."

Patient: "Exactly. "In fact, I am going to do it now."

The patient ran over to the therapist's window and jumped out. The therapist walked to the window and looked down at the street twenty stories below and said: "Splat."

Naturally the highly trained psychoanalysts were skeptical about the therapy provided by counselors with so little training who merely rephrased and parroted what patients told them. However, a good many individuals did seem to benefit from this simplified form of treatment, and it is a technique that is still utilized by many counselors today.

The programs offered by the military will provide helpful information and help veterans reduce the stresses they deal with as they adjust to home after being deployed. Pay serious attention to these programs and utilize the written materials and references provided. They will make things easier for you and your family.

Readjustment to Civilian Life

Having said this, I want to try to provide an explanation of how survival behaviors from the combat area are learned and imprinted into the veteran's mind and how they may be extinguished when he returns home. This isn't complicated. This is information that will make your warrior's (and your) adjustment faster and easier.

You've probably heard of Pavlov's experiment in which he fed dogs and at the same time rang a bell. The dogs associated the bell with food, and soon just ringing the bell would cause them to salivate and their gastric juices to flow. This was called a conditioned response. Psychologists use this mechanism to change behavior. For example, an individual with a germ phobia who goes to a behavioral psychologist might find that the therapist sits with him holding his hands in a bowl of muck. Initially the patient is extremely anxious, as this is his worst fear, but in time as the therapist continues to grasp the patient's hands in the gunk while pointing out that nothing bad has happened, the patient's anxiety diminishes and his brain resets itself. Through this process of what behavioral therapists call "flooding," the patient becomes relaxed.

Let's take a warrior who is in Baghdad, where a suicide bomber sets off an explosion in a crowded market. The warrior associates crowds, Middle Eastern people, baggy clothing, the smells of the market, and loud noises with life-threatening danger. Avoiding crowds, watching people with baggy clothing, being suspicious of Middle Eastern people, reacting to similar odors, and hitting the dirt when he hears loud noises are all protective behaviors, and these behaviors are reinforced as being life-saving behaviors. Now the same veteran returns home and becomes anxious in crowds, around Middle Easterners, seeing people with baggy clothing, smelling those odors, and hearing loud noises. That would seem to be understandable—right?

OK, to dampen these responses, he might want to expose himself to the stimuli that evoke his anxiety. Going to a crowded mall would evoke considerable anxiety initially, but as he stayed in the crowd and nothing harmful happened and as he observed other friendly people walking around safely and as he thought, "I am in the United States and no longer in Baghdad, this place has never been bombed, etc.," his anxiety would gradually diminish. Similarly, he might go to a Middle Eastern restaurant and sit among Middle Easterners until his anxiety fades away. Some combat veterans force themselves to go to fireworks displays to desensitize themselves to the sound of explosions. These are all ways of treating oneself using the flooding technique.

Another approach would be to use stress inoculation training (SIT) in which the warrior gradually exposes himself to crowds by initially sitting in the mall parking lot in his car, then going to the mall when it is nearly empty, and gradually exposes himself to increasing numbers of people. Both flooding and SIT accomplish the same goal. It is the difference between learning to swim by putting your toe in the water and gradually getting in (SIT) versus taking an immediate plunge into the pool (flooding).

Exposure therapy with flooding or stress inoculation can be applied to many of the conditioned behaviors that have developed during deployment. Some behaviors may respond better to other approaches. Let us review the behaviors the warrior has learned through military training and downrange in the combat zone. It is these survival skills that seem abnormal in the civilian setting initially. With time, love, and patience, most warriors are able to let go of these patterns of behavior and adjust to the civilian environment.

The warrior's body responds to stress with the release of adrenaline and noradrenaline, which produce a "flight or fight" reaction. The pupils dilate, breathing and heart rate increase, muscles tense, and the bowels evacuate—all preparing the animal to run or fight. The soldier learns to slow his breathing and focus his attention. He is hyperalert and ready to respond. The body goes through the stages of alarm, resistance, and exhaustion if the stress continues over time.

Poor health, injury, hunger, anger, fatigue, major losses, chemical dependency, lack of coping skills, chronic pain, impulsivity, childhood trauma, repeated abuse, or combat conditions are factors that make the individual more vulnerable to stress and tend to cause the stress reactions to last longer.

Section VI: Normal Reactions to Abnormal Situations and Readjusting to Home

Suppression of Feelings

Your warrior may seem quieter than he used to be. The family may be disappointed that he does not react with jubilation at his homecoming reunion. His seeming withdrawal and lack of emotional expression is likely the result of a number of factors:

- Normal male behavior. Men tend to go to their caves to solve their problems. They have difficulty identifying how they feel and even more problems expressing feelings. One theory is that women learn to soothe themselves as a part of breast-feeding while men stay excited when they express their feelings. Because this lasts so long for men, they avoid the expression of feelings.

- Initial military training where he or she was trained to suppress excitement and fear in order to remain clearheaded in battle.

- Warriors may be quiet as they mentally censor their language and behavior to try to avoid swearing or exhibiting some of the primitive habits they adopted overseas.

- He or she may be suppressing wartime experiences that he or she feels would upset the family or be so foreign to them that they could never understand what the warrior has experienced.

- Soldiers are trained to create an emotional distance from their enemies through the use of impersonal language (targets, KIAs, etc.)

- Emotional detachment from home enables men to function optimally in the field.

- It is impossible to suppress bad feelings without dampening good feelings as well. Fear and anger may be dampened, but joy and pleasure are as well.

This problem will probably solve itself over the next year. In time his or her lizard brain will realize that the warrior is not in the combat zone and recognizing and expressing feelings will not put the veteran in danger. Activities with the family will eventually thaw his or her frozen emotions in most cases. One self-help technique would be to write in detail some of the traumatic experiences the warrior had while deployed. The veteran doesn't have to show anyone what he or she has written. The exercise is designed to help the warrior identify and experience the feelings he or she has about these traumatic experiences. Then the warrior can tear up what has been written and throw it away. Sometimes meeting with buddies he or she served with overseas or other veterans at the VFW will provide an outlet for telling war stories and experiencing some of the feelings the warrior has pushed under the carpet.

Hypervigilance and Startle Reactions

Downrange, hypervigilance is self-protective. Scanning suspicious individuals, piles of material near the road, cars parked nearby, sudden movement, flashes of light, and loud noises are part of the adaptive behaviors soldiers learn in a combat area. Reacting quickly to these triggers is a life-saving reflex as well. These are the reflexes that lead to warriors dropping to the ground when a car backfires, lying down on the front seat of the car when a glass reflects and causes a flash of bright light, attacking a family member who awakens them or comes up behind them, and pulling down the shades so that no one could look into the house. His or her reactions may be triggered by seemingly innocuous stimuli. A variety of situations may precipitate a response: crowds of people, Middle Eastern individuals, violent movies, smells that remind the veteran of war, being closed in, etc. Developing this state of alertness and learning to react without thinking have been protective for the past year. These behaviors won't be dropped in a short period even though they are inappropriate in the civilian setting. They can lead to the warrior withdrawing from social situations where he may encounter a trigger. Again, flooding or stress inoculation approaches can be applied to more quickly overcome these combat habits. The veteran can go to crowded restaurants and resist the temptation to sit in the corner like a gunfighter from the old West. He or she can make him- or herself go to fireworks displays or shooting galleries and desensitize quickly or gradually depending on what he or she feels would be best.

Avoiding Crowds

Warriors are taught in the war zone to avoid crowds that may be attractive to suicide bombers. Similarly they are taught not to bunch up and make themselves targets for the enemy. It is understandable why they might become anxious in crowded areas like the mall at home. Warriors may make themselves go to a crowded mall and flood themselves with the anxiety of the situation all at once or may gradually expose themselves by sitting in the mall parking lot, then approaching the mall on another trip and finally entering the mall for brief periods (toe in the water approach).

A Need for Weapons

Currently soldiers are issued weapons loaded with blanks the second day of BT. They are prepared to defend themselves at all times. Soldiers are never without their weapons in a combat area. They take them to the bathroom. They feel naked and insecure without a means to defend themselves. It is difficult for them to leave their security blankets when they arrive home. It may be difficult for your warrior to be unarmed when he or she first comes home even though, intellectually, the warrior knows it is abnormal for civilians to be walking around with guns. Again, time will overcome this insecurity and habit of being armed. Concern for the children's safety will force him or her to lock up weapons and make sure they are not accessible to the youngsters. Again, locking up weapons or giving them up to other family members for safe keeping will help the veteran get used to walking around unarmed. His or her initial insecurity will diminish as the warrior tells him- or herself that they are in a safe environment. The experiences of being OK without a weapon over time will help diminish the need for it and will build a sense of security. Having said this, I can tell you that most of my Special Forces veteran friends continue to carry. On the other hand, I have taken care of three veterans who were in heavy combat overseas who refused to have anything to do with a weapon after their return. These men described having killed many enemy combatants at relatively close quarters. All were hunters and all gave up this sport after their return. One was a gunsmith who collected and repaired guns prior to his service. He gave away his guns and didn't want to have anything to do with a weapon after he returned.

Defensive Driving

Depending on your warrior's experience overseas, he or she may not want to drive initially. In some assignments soldiers learned to drive at high speeds down the middle of the road to avoid IEDs and ambushes. He or she may be fearful passing under overpasses. The warrior may have the urge to throw a water bottle at cars that approach his or her automobile too closely. Overseas they didn't use seat belts to avoid being trapped in the vehicle. The veteran might have to ride for a while at home until he or she adapts to slower speeds in his or her own lane while driving. As the warrior thinks about where he or she is and observes other people driving on the right side of the road at moderate speeds, he or she will gradually extinguish the life-saving habits developed overseas.

Lack of Self-Restraint

Living in the adverse climatic conditions of Iraq or Afghanistan. Sleeping, eating, and bunking with a primarily male population. Serving in combat. All of these can result in crude and uncivilized behavior. One wife described being awakened by her recently deployed husband to find him urinating in a pop bottle in their bedroom. When she questioned his seemingly bizarre behavior, he said he had done this for a year rather than walk to the privy in the cold of Afghanistan. Similarly, soldiers throughout history have used profane language. In World War I soldiers didn't talk about being killed. They said they were "nipped off of their turd." In Vietnam we used the *f* word so frequently that we inserted it between syllables (un-fucking-believable, fan-fucking-tastic). It is going to take some time and a conscious effort to correct the crude language and habits he or she has developed over the past year. Some veterans may actually have damage to the precortical areas of their brain due to childhood abuse and repeated, severe combat stresses. These brain-damaged warriors may lack the social restraint ordinarily provided by the inhibitory influence of the cortex, resulting in volatile emotional mood swings, increased irritability, impulsiveness, and poor judgment. These veterans will require professional assistance.

Bonding with Other Veterans

The veteran's training and combat experiences have caused the warrior to bond closely with the members of his or her unit. The warrior's life depended on comrades in arms and vice versa. These are some of the closest and most intense relationships he or she has ever experienced. They are like brothers and sisters. It is likely that the veteran will miss these relationships upon return home. Warriors may hang out with comrades who are nearby or go to the VFW to socialize with veterans they know understand their experiences overseas. Speaking the same language and sharing war stories can be healthy and may speed the adaptation to home. It can be also carried to extremes and facilitate a withdrawal from the demands of family life, provide a more comfortable, accepting environment, and retard the warrior's integration into the family. Soldiers, especially under the influence of alcohol or drugs, may fuel each other's anger in an unhealthy way. On the other hand, as we mentioned earlier, the warrior may be comfortable talking with other veterans who understand his or her experiences. Telling stories with other veterans at the VFW may help him or her express suppressed feelings.

Concern for Detail and Intolerance for Error

Attention to detail is life-saving in combat. Making sure that everything is working, that all the supplies and equipment are in place, and that the mission is carried out exactly as planned are all part of staying alive and being successful in combat. Small details like an untied bootlace, a twig snapping, the noise of dog tags clicking together, or dirt in a weapon can lead to disaster not only for the individual but also for the entire unit.

Your veteran may be like Don Corleone in *Godfather I.*
Don Corleone: "I hope you don't mind the way I keep going over this Barzini business.
Michael: No, not at all."
Don Corleone: "It's an old habit. I spent my whole life trying not to be careless. Women and children can afford to be careless, but not men."

Warriors outside of the wire in OIF and OEF focus on the details of soldiering because they know that small errors may lead to injury or death for themselves and their units. They also feel that by developing combat skills and paying attention to the minutiae of their behavior they have some control over their destiny in the field. In the same way, they will at the least shun a comrade who appears to be careless. On the other hand, riding in a vehicle and being hit with an IED or being exposed to a VBIED are situations that are "crap shoots" that are left to chance. In these situations training and skill have little to do with whether they are injured or killed. Because the warrior is so vigilant, he or she may sense conditions that precede danger in the field. Some soldiers said they could "smell" Vietcong in Vietnam. A psychological extension of these efforts to anticipate danger in the combat environment is that of magical thinking. Associating events surrounding an ambush, for example, might lead a unit to the conclusion that eating certain foods or certain weather conditions or performing specific tasks might bring on an attack.

This same control and attention to detail can be annoying to family members at home. These concerns usually fade in time as the warrior's primitive brain begins to accept that he or she will be safe even while more relaxed and less cautious. After I had a heart attack and open-heart surgery I went to cardiac rehabilitation, where I was monitored while carrying out the prescribed exercise program. After a few weeks the staff showed me that what I was doing in rehab was the equivalent of mowing the yard, raking the leaves, or moving furniture at home. Although I agreed with the staff intellectually, I wasn't about to try to do these things at home until, in time, I could see that I wasn't dropping dead and my lizard brain decided it was OK for me to return to a normal level of activity. The same process applies to veterans giving up the patterns of behavior that have kept them alive while deployed. In their heads they agree they no longer need them in civilian life, but it takes time for their primitive brains to accept this and let go of their protective patterns of behavior.

Concern for Safety

For the past year your warrior has been concerned for his or her personal safety as well as the safety of the fellow troops. The veteran has had to anticipate all of the negative events that might occur and take steps to protect against them. The returning warrior brings the same apprehension and concern with him or her when arriving home. He or she may be overly concerned about the safety of family members. The family will likely find this apprehension and concern irrational and unnecessary. The urge by some to carry a weapon is in response to this concern. Patience and understanding on the part of the family and the passage of time will help the veteran let go of his or her apprehension and achieve a realistic view of the family's security.

Physical Complaints

Some troops carry as much as one hundred pounds of equipment and sustain injuries to their backs, knees, and feet and experience aches and pains as a result of this trauma. Also, because of the tendency to suppress and lack of awareness of feelings, depression and other painful emotions may find their expression through somatic complaints. Of course you are going to have the veteran's complaints checked out by the family doctor, but how do you respond when the warrior gripes about his or her head or back hurting, feeling light-headed, stomach being upset, etc.?

1. Listen and try to empathize with his unhappiness and discomfort.
2. Respond with supportive comments such as "It must be difficult to feel that way" or "I'm sorry you are feeling so badly."
3. Try to help him or her come up with ideas. "Is it better when you go for a walk?" "Is it less bothersome when you are distracted?" "Does heat or ice help?"

Section VI: Normal Reactions to Abnormal Situations and Readjusting to Home

4. The key is not to withdraw but to stay engaged and be supportive and encouraging.

Guilt and Sadness

Not all warriors will experience these symptoms but many will. They may feel sadness at leaving their close buddies, sadness for those who were killed or wounded, and guilt for not being wounded or killed themselves (survivor guilt). Some military leaders feel guilty about having ordered men into situations where they were wounded or killed. Some mourn the loss of excitement and the adrenaline rush of battle. I saw a young patient who scheduled an appointment because of symptoms of depression and anxiety. He had five tours in Iraq as a dog handler for a civilian contractor. He trained and utilized dogs to sniff out explosives. When he arrived at the office, he said his depression was gone and he was fine. I asked him what had cured him so quickly. He said, "I just got orders for a sixth tour, Doc, and I can't wait to get back there!" He is now on his fifteenth tour. One of his friends agreed that he was probably an adrenaline junkie, but pointed out that his salary of $17,000 a month was also a motivating factor. (It should be noted his tours were typically a few months in duration.)

Some men have had to order subordinates into situations that resulted in their being killed or injured. Lt. Colonel David Grossman points out that some men experience guilt and remorse for killing an enemy while others do not. Both reactions are normal.

If your warrior suffers from survivor guilt, ask him or her what the deceased buddy would say about the self-criticism. Ask the veteran to imagine what he or she would say if your warrior had died and the comrade had lived. It might help to visit injured buddies who are hospitalized and also the families of pals who were killed.

Make a point to honor those who sacrificed themselves and were wounded or killed in combat.

CMS Huber said Desert Storm raised his mood because the men and women he had trained performed so well in combat during that campaign. He felt good that so few of the soldiers he had been responsible for training were killed or wounded in combat. It is a reminder for officers and NCOs to give themselves credit for the men they trained who performed well and not to focus on those who were killed or wounded, as many tend to do. This is a natural tendency. I used to ask the nurses on the psychiatric unit to give me the names of five patients who came to their minds. Inevitably they named five patients who were particularly difficult and who had relapsed several times. I pointed out that the vast majority of patients recovered and went back to normal lives, but the ones whose names stuck in their minds were the tough cases who weren't doing that well. Officers and NCOs are like these nurses. They think of those trainees who were killed or wounded and forget all of the soldiers who lived because of the skills they taught them.

Complicated Grief

Grief that persists beyond the normal six to nine months is considered complicated grief. The person continues to suffer and is unable to put the loss behind him or her. Symptoms include:

- Continued focus on the loss and memories of the loved one.

- Inability to accept the death of the loved one.

- Extreme longing for the loved one.

- Emotional numbness.

- Uncontrolled crying spells.
- Anhedonia (inability to have fun).
- Prolonged sadness.
- Recurrent emotional dreams about loved one.
- Difficulty carrying out ADLs (activities of daily living).
- Social withdrawal.
- Difficulty forming new close relationships.
- Anger and extreme irritability.
- Lack of trust in others.

How to Help with Mourning and Grief

Mourning is grief out in the open. Everyone grieves, but some people may hold in their feelings. It is healthier to express them in the open and share them with others. You and your spouse both have things to mourn: your identities as you knew each other before deployment; your relationship as it was in the past; his or her comrades lost in battle; and, if he or she was injured, the level of functioning as it was before.

The veteran may have survivor's guilt because he or she is alive and some comrades didn't make it. They may have lost soldiers under their command and feel responsible for their deaths or injury. One approach to help warriors with their guilt is to have them imagine they were the one who died (or was wounded) and the dead buddy was still alive. What would they want their comrade to do? Would they blame others for their death (or injury)? What would they say to a buddy who was alive? Then tell him or her to say these things to him- or herself. Encourage the warrior to visit comrades who are wounded or hospitalized and go with him or her. Accompany him or her to visit the graves and families of buddies who were killed. Injured friends and the families of those who were killed will not blame him or her but will be happy to see their loved one's former comrade and will be grateful that the person took the time to visit them.

Here are some aspects of mourning—the outward expression of grief.

It is OK for men to shed tears. It is the natural response to pain. It is difficult for most men to cry, but it has become more acceptable since Alan Alda started expressing his emotions in the theater. President Clinton did it on cue. Men are physically capable of crying, and they don't have to dress in drag to weep. It helps the healing process. Women have an easier time expressing their emotions, but military training and serving as a soldier may inhibit what can be a useful coping device for the female warrior.

Encourage him or her to talk about the person or thing that you are mourning—how he felt before he or she lost the person or it, and why he or she misses him, her, or the thing.

Encourage him or her to let friends, clergy, and other professionals help. (See Section VIII, which discusses getting a man in for professional help.)

Be patient and encourage your veteran to be patient. Mourning is a healing process that takes time. Visualize the loss as a deep wound that gradually heals.

Encourage warriors to give themselves some slack. Let them express their guilt and recognize that they are human and did the best they could. In the case of survivor guilt, tell the veteran, "Think what you would say if your buddy had survived and you had died. Would you blame him or wish him ill? He feels the same toward you."

Encourage the veteran to ask for help and to let people know what is needed. People who get depressed have a hard time asking for help and a hard time saying no to the demands of others. Have the warrior practice asking others for what he or she needs. Remind the returnee that it makes others feel better to be of help.

Urge the veteran to thank others for helping. When people do help or say something that provides comfort, give them positive feedback.

Encourage veterans to take care of themselves. It seems simple to say they should eat right, exercise, and get checkups, but good health is necessary for feeling good in life. If warriors aren't sleeping and the usual remedies aren't helping, have them see a professional and get back to a restful night's sleep.

Suggest that he or she consider a support group and/or talking to a professional. Therapy is good for everyone. The veteran can always learn things about him- or herself. Talking with peers who understand what the returning warrior is experiencing can be therapeutic.

Tell the vet to listen to the advice of others and then decide what is best. Tell them to trust their own judgment. Some of what they hear will be BS. For example, one widower kept a notebook in his pocket at his wife's funeral. When someone would say, "If there is anything I can do..." he would pull out his notebook and pen and say, "Yes, you can mow the lawn. I'll put you down for Tuesday afternoon." And then he would laugh at the expression on the person's face.

Tell veterans not to rush their feelings. Everyone wants them to move on, get busy, and start socializing, but they may not be ready to do so. Changing their routine will confront them with the fact that things are different and, emotionally, they don't want to face this. They want to turn the clock back and have things the way they were before the loss. Usually people start making themselves get out and do things when they become so lonely they can't stand staying at home by themselves.

Don't go against your natural inclinations. If you tend to withdraw to recharge your batteries then pull in and recharge. If you are an extrovert who gets energy from others then socialize.

Don't make decisions in haste. Most people say wait at least a year before making any big decisions.

Sleep Disturbances

Sleep disturbance is practically a universal problem among returning veterans. Their hypervigilance in the combat zone, the jet lag returning from overseas, the excitement of being home, the adjustment to new surroundings, and the stress and trauma they have experienced all contribute to sleep disturbances and, frequently, nightmares. Most of these difficulties will straighten themselves out on their own in time. Let your warrior nap and sleep if he or she wants. The returning veteran may be able to make up for the sleep he or she has lost if given the opportunity to do so. If other problems such as depression, PTSD, or chemical dependency exist, the sleep problems may persist and serve as an indicator that professional help is needed. If your warrior snores loudly and seems to be gasping for breath, he or she probably suffers from sleep apnea and will benefit from a C-PAP and consultation by a sleep expert. Vivid nightmares respond in many cases to a low dose of Minipress prescribed by a psychiatrist who treats PTSD.

Section VI: Normal Reactions to Abnormal Situations and Readjusting to Home

You can use your Internet search engine to find lists of suggestions for sleep hygiene. Here are a few typical suggestions:

1. Avoid the use of caffeine near bedtime.

2. Avoid vigorous physical activity near bedtime.

3. Don't sleep during the day. (I once had a patient who told me, "Doc, I sleep pretty well at night and in the morning, but in the afternoon I just toss and turn.")

4. Don't eat spicy foods that may cause an upset stomach.

5. Don't watch the clock at night.

6. Use the bed for sleep and sex only. (Don't read, watch television, etc., in bedroom.)

7. Stay awake in bed no longer than fifteen minutes. If you don't get to sleep within this time, get up and do something else until you become sleepy.

8. Use relaxation and distraction to speed the onset of sleep (relax muscles, picture yourself in a peaceful place, count sheep, etc.).

9. Follow a nightly routine.

10. Some find warm milk facilitates sleep.

If this doesn't do the job in terms of getting the veteran to sleep, contact your family physician for a sedative for temporary use until a regular schedule of sleeping at night is established. (Better things for better living through chemistry.)

Excessive Irritability and Anger

Warriors are often sleep-deprived. They had limited hours of sleep in the combat area. They are flown back to the States and experience the jet lag that goes with the flight. The excitement of the reunion with the family may further interfere with their sleep. There may be many demands or perceived demands placed on them by the family when they return. Warriors have had to be careful and exacting in combat. The seeming carelessness of civilian life may be irritating to them. They come home to civilians who may have forgotten about the conflicts in OEF and OIF. The warrior has been facing life-and-death situations and seeing his or her comrades killed or injured. In contrast, civilians appear to be preoccupied with seemingly petty events. Civilians, in general, put themselves before any organization or group. Warriors have been trained and conditioned in combat to put their comrades first. He will likely perceive civilians as being selfish and self-centered. The civilians may offer opinions about the war that are irritating. Veteran warriors may think, "Where were you when I was over there under adverse conditions, defending your freedoms and trying to keep from getting killed?" One soldier told how, after being on duty for sixteen hours, he was awakened for physical exercise in the base camp. Another reported he was given a ticket in the States for driving around the post with his seat belt off. In Iraq he left it off to avoid being trapped in the vehicle, and now he was being punished by an REMF who had no overseas service. Preliminary studies seem to indicate a correlation between the returning veteran's hypervigilance with anger and hostility. TBI and excessive alcohol use appear to correlate as well but not as specifically or directly. Irritability and anger will usually abate in time. Exercise and rest can help speed this process. Use of the heavy and speed bags, meditation, and martial arts are particularly good outlets for anger. Having the warrior write letters to the person(s) who makes him or her angry and then tearing them up can be a way of siphoning off some of the frustration.

A New Program on the Internet

A new online self-management cognitive behavioral therapy treatment program, SM-CBT, is available for veterans with symptoms of PTSD. It has been shown to be effective, inexpensive, accessible, and confidential. The program takes eight weeks, and the positive changes resulting from its use appear to be lasting. Obviously this treatment program offers assistance without stigma. It is self-guided and gives the veteran a feeling of being in control of his treatment.

The Process of Adjusting to a New Identity

Learning about how these behaviors are developed during military training and later in the combat zone will help you understand that they are normal reactions to an abnormal situation. You can see why they are inappropriate in a civilian setting, and you can use flooding or stress inoculation techniques to alter them. At first you will catch yourself *after* you've done the behavior. By paying attention this will progress to *while* you are doing the behavior, and ultimately you will be able to *anticipate* how you used to react and will be able to make the choice to act differently.

Adjustment back to civilian life is a change in identity. You may resist acting differently because you feel that you are a phony and that this isn't you. No it isn't. It is who you want to be. Therefore you have to act like someone else until you assume the new identity. If you go into a hospital setting and see some new student nurses and say "nurse," they don't look up. They don't think of themselves as nurses. They imitate the RNs, and then one day when you say "nurse," they respond—they have the new identity of being a nurse.

It is the same when you are trying to change yourself. You have to pick a civilian you admire and imitate him, and then one day you will have your new civilian identity. "Fake it until you make it," as they say in AA.

Facilitating the Warrior's Adjustment Home

Most veterans adjust to civilian life after serving in combat without professional help. Key to their adjustment is the patience, love, and support of the family, as well as the establishment of a healthy schedule of exercise, healthy diet, sleep, recreation, socialization, and work.

The adaptive behaviors that were developed in the combat zone are no longer necessary, but it will take time for the warrior to let go of them and still feel safe. Some can be sped up by exposure to the phobic situation. For example, a hypervigilant warrior who is upset by seeing a Middle Eastern individual might overcome some of this anxiety by having dinner in a Middle Eastern restaurant surrounded by foreigners. In behavioral therapy this is known as exposure or flooding the individual. For example, a patient with a fear of germs might have therapy where both the patient and the therapist place their hands in a bowl of dirty muck while they discuss the patient's fear of germs. The patient's anxiety is sky high initially but gradually subsides as he realizes nothing terrible has happened. On the other hand, you must judge how anxious your warrior is likely to become. Taking a recently deployed warrior to a shooting range would not be therapeutic if he or she is overwhelmed with anxiety.

Some General Advice

> Even though you are eager to share the experiences your warrior has had while you were apart, you can't completely understand or empathize with what the soldier has been

Section VI: Normal Reactions to Abnormal Situations and Readjusting to Home

through in the combat zone. Just listen supportively to what he or she does say, and be patient and let the warrior take his or her time adjusting.

You might say that you know it was difficult and stressful but that you can never understand fully what the veteran went through or is currently experiencing.

Listen but don't react. If you become upset, it is unlikely that he will continue discussing this topic in the future. For example, if the wife becomes upset when a husband mentions chest pain, he will be unlikely to discuss his chest pain with her in the future.

If you are unable to listen to a topic without becoming upset, tell him that you don't want to hear any more about this situation. You might suggest someone else who could tolerate listening to this particular topic, such as a family member who is a veteran or one of your warrior's comrades in arms.

Be patient and don't push your warrior about talking, emoting, socializing, parenting, or any other activity he or she is reluctant to do. If he or she seems hypervigilant, recognize that this is normal behavior for a combat zone. It took him a year to establish these patterns of behavior, and it will probably take him as long to lose them.

Rest, a good diet, and lots of affection and patience will have a healing effect.

Vigorous exercise by walking, running, swimming, horseback riding, martial arts, weight lifting, heavy bag and speed bag work, etc., can provide an outlet for the warrior's adrenaline.

Two thousand years ago, the Greeks prescribed music and comedies for their melancholic patients. These are still good prescriptions. Soothing, upbeat music is comforting. Listening to and watching comedians is therapeutic. I was leaving my dermatologist's office when he said, "Stay out of the sun." "Why, do I have something that is adversely affected by the sun?" I asked. "No, I say that to all of my patients," he answered. "Don't you psychiatrists have advice you give to all of your patients?" he queried. I thought for a moment and then said, "Don't watch or listen to the news."

Before you decide that your warrior's behavior is pathologic in some way, consult with professionals who have experience with postdeployment adjustment in the military or the VA. If they inform you that the veteran is showing signs of serious problems, such as PTSD, depression, chemical dependency, panic disorder, or some other malady, then you should go ahead and make an appointment for him with his family physician and accompany the returning soldier to the consultation. If it is likely that specialized help is indicated, schedule an appointment with a military medical facility or VA clinic as well.

In this chapter we've discussed how warriors are conditioned by their training and the combat environment to develop patterns of behavior that are necessary for their survival in battle. I've noted that these are normal changes and reactions. They keep these survival behaviors when they return home and, in time, most will gradually give them up as they adjust to civilian life or civilian posting. It is likely that in the neighborhood of 85 percent of veterans will make these adjustments and go on with their lives without professional assistance. We observed that it takes time for the warrior to feel safe at home and to let go what were life-saving behaviors overseas. In the next chapter we'll discuss the 15 percent who continue to have problems. We'll look at some of the common problems seen, their treatment, and also provide some suggestions as to how you may get your loved one to professional help if needed.

Section VII: Pathological Problems

Chapter Six: PTSD, Depression, Survival Guilt, Food Addiction, Chemical Dependency, Sex Addiction, Gambling, Internet Addiction.

Getting the Veteran to Treatment

In my book *Loving a Depressed Man*, I discuss the reasons depressed men are more difficult to identify and treat:

"Men are less likely to seek help from caregivers and, because of their tendency to try to solve their own problems, males tend to self-medicate, hide their feelings, or rely on compulsive activities to relieve their depressive illnesses. They have difficulty recognizing or expressing their feelings. They tend to act out with irritability and anger rather than introspection and sadness when they become depressed. As a result, they present as having problems with alcohol, anger management, gambling, sexual indiscretion, or throwing themselves into work; some have physical complaints. They act out in self-destructive ways rather than expressing their feelings of hopelessness. A number of sociological, psychological, and biological factors are behind these phenomena. John Gray in his popular book Men Are from Mars, Women Are from Venus, *observes that men use language to express thoughts and ideas while women use words to convey emotions. John Lynch, PhD, and Christopher Kilmartin, authors of* The Pain Behind the Mask, *note that fathers are typically distant from a family; the primary caregiver is usually the mother. As a result, instead of identifying with the mother like girls, young boys form an identity*

on what the mother is not, or an antifeminine model. They imagine that the distant father is strong, rational, competitive, dominant, and restricted emotionally. They find models for masculinity in movie heroes like John Wayne, Clint Eastwood, Charles Bronson, Chuck Norris, Steven Segal, Bruce Willis, and Vin Diesel. They want intimacy with their caregiver mothers but fear being engulfed or being labeled "mama's boys." They push away from their mothers but fear abandonment. Because of these influences, many men have difficulty admitting vulnerability—which they see as a sign of weakness. They struggle to recognize their feelings and, when asked how they feel, answer with their thoughts instead. Sometimes a male patient will ask me to tell him how he feels. I place my hands on both sides of my head, lean down, shut my eyes, and say, 'There's a woman in the front row with a watch.' The patient usually gets it—I am not a mind reader."

Add to these factors a legacy of General Patton's concept of mental health, and you can see why your (male) warrior will probably be resistant to the idea of seeking help. Women are better at recognizing and expressing their feelings and also about seeking and accepting assistance, although military women may be more resistant than civilian females because of their training and experience. The military culture thinks of itself as self-sufficient, and asking for help implies they can't make it on their own. Of the returning OIF veterans who said they were in need of help, only 40 percent actually contacted a mental health professional. Some active-duty types worry about their security clearances as well. In my private psychiatric practice, I see a number of career soldiers who come to me because they do not want references to psychiatric care in their medical record.

One approach to helping a soldier consult with a professional is to focus on the physical complaints he or she has that are associated with the psychiatric problems. For example, convince the person to go to the family physician for help with problems sleeping or, if applicable, stomach problems. You can alert your doctor's nurse of the problems you are seeing so she can brief the physician in advance. In addition, you might solicit the aid of other veterans to talk with your warrior about seeking help. You may want to mention that one of the veteran's benefits is care with the VA and that he or she might be eligible to receive medication and possibly disability benefits for the symptoms that have developed since returning from deployment. If the family doctor has any influence with the veteran, he may be able to persuade the patient to take advantage of VA benefits by going to the VA for an evaluation with a mental health professional.

Post-Traumatic Stress Disorder (PTSD)

There have always been psychological and physiological reactions to the adverse conditions of combat. Napoleon's chief medical officer, Dominique Larrey, treated nostalgia with a program featuring music and exercise. "Nostalgia," "soldier's heart," and "Da Costa's syndrome" were the terms used in the Civil War. "Shell shock" and "effort syndrome" were the World War I terms. Thomas Salmon, surgeon general of the army, observed that illness, particularly shell shock, provided an honorable excuse to leave the field of battle. After being evacuated it was necessary for the victims of shell shock to maintain their symptoms to avoid seeing themselves as cowards. Salmon developed the four principles of military psychiatry: 1. Proximity—treat psychiatric casualties close to the battle area (within the sounds of the guns). 2. Simplicity—treat with rest, food, and a shower. 3. Immediacy—begin treatment at once. 4. Expectancy—assure the soldier that he would soon return to his unit. Many supposed victims of gas attacks turned out to be suffering from psychological stress reactions during the trench warfare. After World War I, there were nearly nine thousand soldiers receiving disability checks for "functional disease of the heart," which we now classify as an anxiety disorder. Psychiatry during World War II was dominated by psychoanalysis in the United States. Brigadier General William Menninger was in charge of psychiatry in the army and later was president of the American Psychiatric Association. Psychoanalysis taught that everyone was on a continuum between mental health and mental illness and the degree of pathology you had at any one time was a reflection of one's ability to cope with internal anxiety and stress. Karl Menninger described this in his book *The Vital Balance*. Franz Alexander, who founded the Chicago Psychoanalytic Institute, wrote that many supposed physical illnesses were manifestations of unconscious conflicts. Asthma was, for example, "the cry for the mother." The military adopted this approach and described how soldiers with gastrointestinal complaints "lacked the stomach for war." (As an aside, Jules Masserman wrote a paper as a joke about this time describing the ingrown toenail as anger turned on the self. To his surprise, many analysts complimented him on his insight and courage in writing about this neglected topic.) It was observed that men in combat long enough and under enough stress would begin to show symptoms of "battle fatigue" no matter how strong or healthy they were prior to their exposure to battle. The intensity of combat, length of exposure, and the leadership and quality of social supports in the unit influenced the ability of the soldier to withstand stress. The average soldier's breaking point was eighty-eight (not necessarily consecutive) days during which the soldier's unit suffered casualties. Cohesive units with good leaders had fewer psychiatric casualties and soldiers who endured combat stress longer without breaking down. The saying was that "Even Jack Armstrong would show symptoms if he was in combat long enough." It took some time for Salmon's principles from World War I to be discovered and reinstituted. When they were, psychiatrists were assigned to combat divisions, and Salmon's methods (similar to Dominique Larrey's) were put into place with positive results. In World War II, Captain Fred Hanson in the First Infantry Division showed he could return more than 70 percent of battle fatigue casualties to their combat units with forty-eight hours of rest in forward areas. Soldiers who presented with symptoms of battle-induced stress in Korea were diagnosed with combat stress reactions and were immediately treated using Salmon's principles. Colonel Albert J. Glass used battalion surgeons and medics to carry out his forward treatment of psychiatric casualties. In addition soldiers in combat units were rotated out of Korea after nine months, and all soldiers in Korea received at least two weeks of R&R (rest and recuperation) during their tours of duty. As a result, psychiatric casualties in Korea were low, and 90 percent of soldiers with combat stress were returned to duty. In Vietnam we described soldiers who broke down in combat as suffering from "combat stress" or "gross stress reactions." Like Colonel Glass in Korea, we instituted Salmon's principles immediately. We reported a low incidence of combat stress reactions and a high incidence of those being returned to duty. However, we soon learned that large numbers of troops suffered from chemical dependency problems and that race relations in the units were a huge problem. Another psychiatric problem in Vietnam was the soldiers who were inducted as part of Project 100,000, a plan devised by Secretary of Defense Robert McNamara as a part of President Johnson's War on Poverty. Social planners of the Great Society in 1966 conceived a plan to fill the military ranks and to help impoverished, intellectually challenged men (half had IQs below eighty-five, and some had IQs as low as sixty-two) by permitting them to enter military service. This plan led to misery and death for a good many of them. Put simply, one hundred thousand men who failed to meet induction intelligence standards would be permitted to enlist or would be drafted each year. They were to undergo remedial training like the STEP soldiers had received. Unfortunately, by the time the program was started, there were no remedial programs in place for these men, and they essentially went through the training that every soldier was given. Forty percent of these men were black. Blacks comprised 12 percent of the military as a whole. The majority came from urban ghetto environments. Black activists saw the project as a means to weaken the black power movement in the United States. The plan was that military service would provide these individuals with income, training, and experience in soft skills fields. They would work in food service, wire communications, and supply jobs that did not require extensive technical training and that might later have civilian counterparts. It was hoped that many would find a career in the military while others would be able to use their military experience and training to obtain work in the civilian job force. The health and educational benefits would also be of help to them in their future lives. Psychologically, military service would raise their self-esteem and self-confidence. Unfortunately the idealistic ideas leading to the conception of this program were not shared by the military organization. The first two numbers of the "New Standards" men's service numbers were 67 and 68. For the 48 percent who enlisted, their serial number began with RA 67 or RA 68, and the 46 percent who were drafted had serial numbers that began with US 67 or US 68. In either case, they were easily identified as having been inducted with low AFQT scores. Later, serial numbers were dropped and Social Security numbers were used instead, which provided some anonymity for the Project 100,000 participants. The group was cruelly referred to as "McNamara's Morons." McNamara himself referred to the group as the "subterranean poor." They were frequently recycled in basic training and scapegoated by their units. In addition to their intellectual limitations, their coping skills were less than average. Military psychiatrists during the Vietnam era noted that this was a high-risk group. Although the plan was to train them for duties in support units, 140,000 of these men were trained for combat units. Fifty percent of the New Standards men were assigned to combat in the marines. They were killed at over twice the rate of other soldiers. One commanding officer said disparagingly, "They were so dumb in the field that when you told them to get down, they started boogying!" A classic paper by two military psychiatrists in Vietnam, Crowe and Colbach, noted that 30 percent of the Project 100,000 soldiers were referred to psychiatry during a six-month period as opposed to 2.8 percent of nonproject men. In other words, the ratio was ten project soldiers for every one nonproject soldier being sent to mental health facilities at Qui Nhon. In addition, Project 100,000 soldiers were referred for ineffectiveness twice as frequently as nonproject soldiers. In Crowe and Colbach's sample, 12 percent of the project soldiers were referred for administrative discharge because of ineffectiveness during a six-month period, and it was projected that nearly one-fourth of the project soldiers would be deemed ineffective over a one-year period. During the Vietnam War, over two million men were drafted, and of these, 563,000 received less than honorable discharges, 529,000 were administratively discharged, and 34,000 were imprisoned following court-martial convictions. Many who were discharged under less than honorable conditions were not entitled to the benefits that most veterans receive after military service. In the 1980s it was noted that the New Standards men were reassigned eleven times greater than their peers, and somewhere between 9 and 22 percent had remedial training. The all-volunteer force was instituted in 1973. Military organization, training, and leadership were revised to enhance unit cohesion as a way to increase resistance to combat stress. Psychiatric consultation regarding these changes was not sought by higher command. Military psychiatrists did begin consultation programs with commanders, and outreach programs for field units were developed. During the Persian Gulf War, some combat stress control teams consulted with line units. Their posttrauma reviews included suggestions to command as to how the leaders might manage the troops postdeployment to hopefully reduce the incidence of PTSD. Post-traumatic stress is a diagnosis developed by a group of psychiatrists in 1980 to describe a constellation of symptoms exhibited by veterans following their service Vietnam. It was applied to civilian victims who were exposed to extreme trauma as well. A recent RAND Corporation study found that nearly one in five—18.5 percent—of veterans returning from OIF and OEF exhibited symptoms of PTSD or some form of major depression. As of December 2008, four thousand troops had been killed and over thirty thousand returned with visible wounds and a range of permanent disabilities. Colonel Charles W. Hoge, in his book *Once a Warrior—Always a Warrior*, observes that men and women who show stress reactions in battle seldom go on to later develop PTSD. He feels these are two separate entities and that PTSD is the extension of the behaviors men develop and utilize to cope with the stressful combat environment.

Diagnoses in psychiatry are descriptive and based on historical and observational evidence. The Diagnostic and Statistical Manuals were an outgrowth of Brigadier General William Menninger's 1943 "Medical 203," a War Department technical bulletin. Psychiatrists described the symptoms of PTSD and entered them into the Diagnostic and Statistical Manual III in 1980, and the condition became an illness, in the same way they deleted homosexuality from the manual in 1973 and it no longer was considered an illness. "Neurosis," a once-popular psychiatric diagnosis, was eliminated as well.

No other medical specialty produces and eliminates diagnoses in this manner. It should be noted that when we are able to diagnose the actual physical basis for mental illnesses with laboratory, genetic, or radiological testing of some type, the diagnoses will again be revised. Proton emission tomography (PET) scans, for example, may lead to more specific diagnoses of PTSD in the near future. Recently blood tests have been developed that assist in making an objective diagnosis of traumatic brain injury (TBI).

The diagnosis of a mental disorder may not reflect disability. During the initial stages of World War II, psychiatrists were placed in the induction centers, where they used a lengthy questionnaire developed by Harry Stack Sullivan to screen out "neurotics." Lou Wessalius, MD, was a consultant at the Menninger Clinic when I was a resident there. He described how boring the work in the induction center was for him. All day long he would read the lengthy questionnaire to one young man after another. Some were malingerers who wanted to avoid military service. Dr. Wessalius said that it was obvious one fellow was trying to answer all of the questions incorrectly, and he thought he would have a little fun with him.

Dr. Wessalius: "Where does bacon come from?"
Inductee: "A sheep."
Dr. Wessalius: "No, try again."
Inductee: "A cow."
Dr. Wessalius: "No, try again."
Inductee: "A goat."
Dr. Wessalius: "No, try again."
(The inductee realized the psychiatrist wasn't going to let him off this question until he got it right. He sighed and sat back in his chair.)
Inductee: "A pig."
Dr. Wessalius: "No, try again."
The inductee's eyes opened wide with surprise as he stared open-mouthed, wondering if he was indeed mentally ill.

More than a division a month were being excluded from duty at the induction centers. The military feared it would not be able to muster an army if this trend continued. The word came down to stop eliminating neurotics, and those who had been excluded were declared fit for duty. A subsequent study showed that the so-called neurotics actually did better in combat than those who were considered normal during the previous screening. One theory was that individuals with free-floating anxiety felt better when they knew the source of their fears (the enemy) and could do something about it (shoot back). World War II coined the terms "combat exhaustion" and "battle fatigue." It was observed that everyone, given enough stress for a long enough period, would develop symptoms of stress in the battle zone. On one of the Pacific islands during WWII, physicians were forbidden to evacuate psychiatric casualties.

A subsequent study showed that while soldiers with psychiatric diagnoses were not evacuated for a time, the number of evacuees with concussion injuries increased proportionally. In Vietnam, if a unit wanted us to evacuate an individual for his safety or the safety of his unit, we found a way and a diagnosis to expedite the wishes because we knew he would not survive if we didn't get him out of there. In Korea and Vietnam, we used "acute combat stress reaction" and "gross stress reaction," and—as noted earlier—it was not until 1980 that post-traumatic stress disorder became an official diagnosis. OIF and OEF have reported a large number of soldiers with traumatic brain injury (TBI). Colonel Hoge, in *Once a Warrior—Always a Warrior*, notes that many of these cases are really concussion injuries or minimal traumatic brain injuries (mTBI) and that many individuals prefer this diagnosis to a more psychological-sounding disability such as PTSD. Dr. Hoge also notes, and I concur, that symptoms arising in the combat zone are, in many cases, normal reactions to an abnormal situation. In the same way, Dr. Hoge sees the symptoms of post-traumatic stress disorder as the adaptive and stress-related behaviors that warriors develop in a combat zone that are carried over to the postdeployment stage and are inappropriate in civilian life.

Criteria for the Diagnosis of PTSD

The original criteria in the American Psychiatric Association's DSM III in 1980 were further revised in DSM-IV-R in 2000.

    A. Stressor

        The person has been exposed to a traumatic event in which both of the following have been present:

    1. The person has experienced, witnessed, or been confronted with an event or events that involve actual or threatened

death or serious injury, or a threat to the physical integrity of oneself or others.

2. The person's response involved intense fear, helplessness, or horror.

B. Intrusive Recollection

The traumatic event is persistently reexperienced in at least one of the following ways:

1. Recurrent and intrusive distressing recollections of the event, including images, thoughts, or perceptions.

2. Recurrent distressing dreams of the events.

3. Acting or feeling as if the traumatic event were recurring (includes a sense of reliving the experience, illusions, hallucinations, and dissociative flashback episodes, including those that occur upon awakening or when intoxicated).

4. Intense psychological distress at exposure to internal or external cues that symbolize or resemble an aspect of the traumatic event.

5. Physiological reactivity upon exposure to internal or external cues that symbolize or resemble an aspect of the traumatic event.

C. Avoidant/numbing

Persistent avoidance of stimuli associated with the trauma and numbing of general responsiveness (not present before the trauma), as indicated by at least three of the following:

1. Efforts to avoid thought, feelings, or conversations associated with the trauma.

2. Efforts to avoid activities, places, or people that arouse recollections of the trauma.

3. Inability to recall an important aspect of the trauma.

4. Markedly diminished interest or participation in significant activities.

5. Feeling of detachment or estrangement from others.

6. Restricted range of affect (i.e., unable to have loving feelings).

7. Sense of foreshortened future (i.e., doesn't expect to have a career, marriage, children, or a normal life span).

   i. Hyperarousal

   Persistent symptoms of increasing arousal (not present before the trauma) indicated by at least two of the following:

1. Difficulty falling or staying asleep.

2. Irritability or outbursts of anger.

3. Difficulty concentrating.

4. Hypervigilance.

5. Exaggerated startle response.

D. Duration

> Duration of the disturbance (symptoms in B, C, and D) is more than one month.

E. Functional Significance

> The disturbance causes clinically significant distress or impairment in social, occupational, or other important areas of functioning.
>
> Specify if:
>
> Acute: Duration of symptoms less than three months. Chronic: If duration of symptoms is three months or more.
>
> Specify if:
>
> With or without delay onset: Onset of symptoms at least six months after the stressor.

DREAMS is a mnemonic to remember the symptoms of PTSD once a trauma history has been obtained.

D=Detachment (alexithymia) from the event or in relationships with others. It may be manifest as a general numbing of emotional responsiveness.

R=Reexperiencing the event in the form of nightmares, recollections, or flashbacks.

E=Event had emotional effects. The event involved substantial emotional distress, with threatened death, loss of physical integrity, and feelings of helplessness or disabling fear.

A=Avoidance. The patient avoids places, activities, or people that remind him or her of the event.

M=Month in duration. The symptoms have been present for longer than one month.

S=Sympathetic hyperactivity or hypervigilance. Sympathetic hyperactivity or hypervigilance, which may include insomnia, irritability, and difficulty concentrating.

Positron emission tomography (PET) scans of the brain have identified parts of the limbic system (the primitive "lizard brain"), particularly the amygdala and the hippocampus, to be involved in individuals with PTSD. There is a loss of volume of the hippocampus.

The VA sends this self-administered form to all veterans after their return from combat service in Iraq or Afghanistan. Here is an abbreviated form of that screening tool.

PTSD SCREEN FOR WAR VETERANS (*Source: US Department of Veterans Affairs Afghan & Iraq Post-Deployment Screen, Attachment B. Screening for risk factors associated with development of post-traumatic stress disorder (PTSD).*)

Have you ever had any experience that was so frightening, horrible, or upsetting that in the past month you...

1. Have had nightmares about it or thought about it when you didn't want to?

    YES NO

2. Tried hard not to think about it or went out of your way to avoid situations that reminded you of it?

    YES NO

3. Were constantly on guard, watchful, or easily startled?

    YES NO

4. Felt numb or detached from others, activities, or your surroundings?

    YES NO

PTSD is a physical illness. Some individuals feel that traumatic brain injury is a physical—and therefore more legitimate—injury than PTSD. This is incorrect. PTS. causes organic (physical) alterations in the brain as well. The changes in the brain occurring in PTSD can be identified with medical tests. As noted earlier, positron emission tomography (PET) scans of the brain have identified parts of the limbic system (the primitive "lizard brain"), particularly the amygdala and the hippocampus, to be involved in individuals with PTSD. There is a loss of volume of the hippocampus. Recently these scans have been able to diagnose PTSD with 95 percent accuracy. Chronic stress may damage the prefrontal cortex and weaken the individual's ability to inhibit his impulses as well as his responses to stress. Childhood trauma, mental problems in the family, limited social support, preexisting psychological problems, limited coping skills and, especially among female soldiers, sexual abuse, may predispose to PTSD and also make recovery more difficult.

It is easy to see how soldiers in a combat zone would show what are described as the symptoms of PTSD. Warriors who are exposed to life-threatening events in battle (A) have the experience of time slowing down and the ability to recall minute details of the situation. Vasopressin is released in the brain, which imprints the memory and details of the event in the brain (this occurs at the time of any peak experience). These memories are stored in the hippocampus of the brain and can be evoked by exposure to stimuli that trigger memories of these traumatic experiences as flashbacks. There may be a period of exhaustion and numbing of emotions and suppression of memories right after battle contact and later a return of (B) intrusive recollections of the traumatic events. These memories evoke the uncomfortable, frightening fight-or-flight reactions experienced at the time of the event, and the individual makes an effort to avoid cues associated with the trauma (C) and to suppress his feelings. He may withdraw in an effort to avoid stimuli. He avoided thinking about his future in order to focus on the mission. Thoughts of the future were accompanied by concerns for his personal safety, which interfered with optimal functioning in the field. Under stress the individual's adrenaline is flowing, which causes him to be ready to run or to fight. He is hyperalert, requires less sleep, is more irritable, and is ready to move quickly at a moment's notice (D). While criterion A implies that there must be a specific, identifiable event, so-called "support troops" in OEF and OIF live in adverse conditions under constant threats of death and injury. They are susceptible to symptoms of PTSD as a result of their constant exposure to life-threatening stress even though they aren't kicking in doors or shooting people. For example, living in fear of an IED or a VBIED for a month may be as stressful as a single exposure to an explosive device. Recently the military and the VA have changed their criteria for diagnosing PTSD. Instead of requiring documentation of a specific traumatic event triggering the illness, they now acknowledge that the accumulative effect of a number of stressors may lead to the diagnosis as well.

A variety of treatments are proposed for PTSD, which suggests that there isn't one successful recommended approach for this disorder. The four programs that appear to be most effective for the treatment of PTSD are exposure therapy, cognitive therapy, stress inoculation, and eye movement desensitization and reprocessing. Medication may provide some help as well. Below are descriptions of some of the approaches that may be utilized by the professional you and your warrior contact for assistance.

Cognitive Behavioral Therapy (CBT)

This popular, effective approach focuses on behavioral techniques as well as changing negative thought processes to positive. Flooding and stress inoculation described in the previous section are CBT techniques. This program was tried on the Internet, and 25 percent of the veterans who had been diagnosed with PTSD who used it were relieved of their symptoms. This has generated great interest because it would be easy to make it available to veterans even in rural areas, it does not make many demands on professional staff time, and it appears to be as effective as any approach currently available. Various approaches are utilized, including journaling detailed accounts of the traumatic event that was sustained. The therapist may identify "stuck points" where the warrior feels he was worthless because he didn't save his buddy, for example, and challenge his beliefs by asking what anyone else would have done under the same circumstances. What would he have said had he been the buddy and the buddy been him? A medic who blamed himself for the death of his buddy in the field was confronted with the fact that he put in a chest tube, intravenous fluids, and a tracheostomy while under fire. The therapist noted that a chest surgeon could not have done more but would have known it. The therapist also noted that you couldn't get a chest surgeon to crawl out under fire to administer emergency care.

Virtual Reality/Flooding

Using modern technology, soldiers are put into the battle situation and reexperience the trauma that led to their difficulties. As these exposures are repeated, the flight-or-fight response to the situation is weakened. This is a modern version of the sodium amytal interviews that Roy R. Grinker employed during World War II. We carried out a few of these at Fort Knox with returning Vietnam veterans and again in Vietnam in the First Infantry Division. Men were given intravenous sodium amytal and asked to count backward until they began to slur their speech. Then we asked them to recount their traumatic combat experiences in detail as if they were there. These sessions were usually quite dramatic with the soldier patients screaming, sobbing, and expressing murderous rage. Those with hysterical paralysis, blindness, muteness, etc., were instantly "cured" using this technique and with the promise of a thirty-day pass when they recovered. However, like Grinker's results, any attempt to return them to the field resulted in an immediate reoccurrence of their maladies.

At Fort Knox and again in Vietnam, we discovered we didn't really need the sodium amytal to achieve the same results. Our social work/psychology technicians could talk with our patients and relieve their hysterical symptoms in a fairly brief period. The techs provided a shower, rest, hot food, kindness, and empathy, and symptom relief was rewarded while failure to recover was not. For example, patients at Fort Knox were told that once they recovered they would receive a thirty-day pass while, if they failed to respond to treatment, they would be retained in the hospital for further evaluation and treatment. We had a 100 percent recovery rate. In

Vietnam men were told that their experience of paralysis in the field was a fairly normal reaction. We explained that unconsciously their brain was telling them to run from this life-threatening situation, and yet they also knew that they would be in serious trouble if they actually ran. Their subconscious solved the problem by making them paralyzed, which got them out of danger but in a way that they would not be punished. They were told that with an opportunity to ventilate, rest, and exercise, they would soon be up and about. We indicated that they would not be returning to the field and that they could anticipate getting stronger and stronger as they exercised. One hundred percent of these cases also recovered. Of those we initially attempted to return to the field, 100 percent relapsed.

Eye Movement Desensitization and Reprocessing (EMDR) Therapy

Supposedly the memories in PTSD are improperly stored in the brain and are, through EMDR, connected with other networks in the brain. Negative concepts are corrected. Andrew Solomon, in his book *Noonday Demon: An Atlas of Depression,* says, "While many therapies—psychoanalysis, for example—comprise beautiful theories and limited results, EMDR has silly theories and excellent results." As Solomon eloquently notes, it is difficult to understand why EMDR works, but the reported results with PTSD are positive. Veterans are asked to recount traumatic experiences and negative thoughts or feelings associated with the memories. At the same time, they engage in bilateral stimulation, such as rapid eye movements. Alternative evaluations of the traumatic experiences and the negative memories are proposed, and the eye movements are repeated.

Medicine

Medications are prescribed for PTSD, but in my opinion they have limited success. Zoloft is a selective serotonin reuptake inhibitor (SSRI). It is the only medication that is FDA approved for the treatment of chronic PTSD. Paxil is another SSRI that is approved for the treatment of acute PTSD. The other SSRIs (Prozac, Lexapro, Celexa, Luvox) have been shown to be helpful. In addition, the older first- and second-generation tricyclic antidepressants (Elavil, Tofranil, Anafranil, Norpramine, Aventyl, Pamelor, Vivactil) as well as the monomine oxidase inhibitors (Nardil, Parnate, Marplan) have been noted to show some effectiveness as well. Minor tranquilizers, typically the benzodiazepines (Xanax, Ativan, Klonopin), and the older ones (Valium, Librium Atarax) are used as Band-Aids to try to control the individual's anxiety. In some cases major tranquilizers like the newer atypicals (Zyprexa, Seroquel, Risperdal, Abilify, Fanapt, Saphyris) and the older ones (Thorazine, Mellaril, Stellazine, Prolixin, Navane, Haldol) have been used as adjunctive therapy. Sleeping medications (Ambien, Lunesta, Restoril, Dalmane) or a sedative antidepressant (Desyrel) are used to help the individual get back on a normal sleep cycle. Beta blockers given shortly after the traumatic experience have been shown to reduce the incidence of PTSD later on. The alpha-adrenergic antagonist prazosin (Minipress), commonly prescribed for hypertension, has been shown to improve the sleep of PTSD patients. Minipress is also used to quell vivid nightmares. The nightmares described by veterans are frequently extremely vivid. One veteran said he had dreams of being a sniper and an assassin that were so detailed and real that he logged the odometer on his automobile to assure himself he hadn't killed someone during the night.

Dream Revision Techniques (or Imagery Rehearsal Therapy, or IRT)

1. State or write down the content of the nightmare.

2. Rescript the nightmare to give it a positive ending.

3. Memorize the revised nightmare by repeating it over and over to yourself or a confidant or into a recording device.

4. Go to sleep and observe the outcome.

One advantage of IRT or dream revision is that the patient does not have to go over the actual trauma but rather the symbolic material in the dream itself. It is possible to change the metaphor without revisiting the stressful experience.

Relaxation Techniques

Dr. Robert T. London, MD, described his success using behavioral modification techniques such as reciprocal inhibition and systematic desensitization along with guided imagery in his treatment of PTSD. Dr. London uses cognitive therapy to prevent these stress-related disorders. He teaches techniques that avoid "all or nothing" thinking or the pitfalls of "this or that" type of thoughts. He uses the idea of possibilities and probabilities, where everything is possible but the real probabilities are detailed. For example, a soldier might be killed overseas, but he might also win the lottery. The probability lies somewhere in between.

Group Therapy

Group therapy is a helpful, effective approach in the military. Military training has bonded men to one another in their units, and it is this affection for comrades that sustains men in battle. It is natural for returning veterans to turn to one another for support in veterans organizations and in therapy as well. It is important, however, that the group be structured and led by a professional. This professional could be a warrior who has made a successful adjustment after deployment and who has been trained in group therapy techniques to help veterans suffering from PTSD. Without the guidance of a trained caregiver, the group members may avoid common painful topics and may focus their anger on scapegoat targets rather than looking at what is really bothering each of them. For example, during Vietnam a group of waiting wives formed a local support group in a civilian setting. They supported one another with the difficulties inherent in their roles as single parents living and working in a civilian setting. They shared their concerns for the safety of their spouses serving in Vietnam until one of the husbands was killed in action. This event was so upsetting to the group members that they asked the new widow to leave the group. Had they had a professional leader, they could have provided sympathy and support for the woman who lost her husband and been able to work through their fears that their husbands might meet a similar fate.

Conventional Psychotherapy

An important factor for success with any psychotherapeutic approach is to have a therapist to whom the patient can relate. If the therapist has military and/or combat experience, this would be a plus. If the counselor has worked with veterans and their families, this would also make it easier for the patient to relate to him. It is important for the therapist to remain with the patient over time and to listen to him in a nonjudgmental manner. Once the patient is able to talk openly with the therapist, identify and express his feelings, and share the traumatic experiences that trouble him, his symptoms will likely diminish over time. Survivor guilt, mourning the loss of comrades in arms, and anger management are some of the problems that may be helped with conventional therapy. This approach might be of help as an adjunctive treatment to deal with the childhood trauma and other predisposing and aggravating factors that contribute to the development of PTSD.

Alaskan Native American Treatment and Pet Therapy

I mention these unusual approaches because they are in the literature and because they illustrate the wide variety of approaches still being used for the treatment of PTSD. The Alaskan holistic approach involves talking circles, sweat houses, and substance hunts. Providing dogs to veterans with PTSD has been shown to be therapeutic, as the dogs provide unconditional love and companionship that is tolerated by the warriors.

Generalized Anxiety Disorder (GAD)

Command Sergeant Major Gary Huber noted that there is a CD available online that is used by army chaplains to help soldiers reduce their anxiety and relax. You can click on it at http://copingstratagiescd.com. It provides some relaxation exercises that are beneficial to anyone, but particularly men who have experienced combat stress.

Depression

Clinical depression frequently accompanies PTSD in veterans during postdeployment. Women receive this diagnosis twice as often as men, but it appears to the author that this is a false statistic. Men typically engage in compulsive behaviors in an effort to solve their own problems. They don't present with depression but rather as workaholics, alcoholics, drug abusers, gamblers, food addiction, Internet addicts, sex addicts, etc. In the military, depression is often overlooked once the diagnosis of PTSD is made. This is easy to do. PTSD and depression have a number of symptoms in common, including sleep disturbance, preoccupation with the present and past and inability to visualize the future, increased irritability, impaired concentration, social withdrawal, anhedonia, difficulty making decisions, obsessive rumination and preoccupation with negative events, and a limitation of functioning due to either disability. For a detailed discussion of how to understand and help a depressed man, see my book *Loving a Depressed Man*.

It is important to recognize that both are present if they are because treatment is a little different for each. In addition, if either is present and not observed by the caregivers, the response to treatment for the other condition is likely to be compromised.

The symptoms of depression are:

- Sleep disturbance, usually with early morning awakening, but some people have hypersomnia and stay in bed much of the time. Those who overeat, oversleep, and feel worse as the day goes on are referred to as having atypical depression.

- Appetite disturbance, usually with weight loss, but some overeat.

- Difficulty concentrating. This may be mistaken for a memory problem.

- Typically depressed individuals feel worse in the morning and better as the day goes on (except for those with atypical depression).

- Loss of energy. Everything is an effort, and the depressed veteran has to push himself to carry out the simplest tasks (inertia).

- Things that were pleasurable are no longer enjoyable (anhedonia).

- It is an effort to smile and be out around others, and so the individual avoids social events, doesn't want to answer the phone, and withdraws from life (social withdrawal).

- There is a tendency to be preoccupied with the negative aspects of the present and past and to be unable to see the future (negative rumination). This symptom is stressful for caregivers because the individual stiff-arms any efforts to cheer him up and magnifies and dwells on any slightly negative comment.

- Difficulty making decisions. This is why the caregiver needs to go ahead and make appointments and decisions for the depressed individual.

- Loss of libido. Depressed men may have sex as often as usual, but it is not as pleasurable for them.

- Crying spells. A very embarrassing symptom for a macho man.

- Irrational guilt.

- Feelings of hopelessness and helplessness.

- Feeling like pulling the covers over his head and shutting out the world.

- Thinking of running away or giving up.

- Suicidal ideation.

The Greeks described these symptoms in 500 BC. They thought an excess of black bile caused the illness, and they named it melan (black) cholia (bile), or melancholy. Individuals were recognized in the Middle Ages who had these symptoms. For a while demons were thought to have caused them, and drills were used to get rid of the demons. More recently the Freudian idea was that depression was caused by anger turned on the self, and patients were asked to beat rugs and chop wood to get rid of their angry feelings. In 1970 it was possible to measure neurotransmitters in the brain, and three findings known as the biogenic amine hypothesis were:

1. Norepinephrine and serotonin were low in the brains of depressed patients.

2. You could produce symptoms of depression by giving a drug (i.e., Reserpine) that lowered norepinephrine and serotonin in the brain.

3. We had some antidepressants that were accidentally discovered before 1970, and any drug that had an antidepressant effect also raised the levels of norepinephrine and serotonin.

The biogenic amine hypothesis was translated into the term "chemical imbalance," and everyone stopped talking about their analysts and started referring to their chemical imbalances at cocktail parties. These findings, together with the introduction of lithium as a mood stabilizer for bipolar disorder, caused the pendulum in psychiatry to shift from psychology to psychopharmacology. Prior to 1970, psychoanalysts argued that antidepressants were mood elevators and major tranquilizers were chemical straitjackets. They felt the only way to get to the root of mental illness was through psychoanalysis. Lithium was a naturally occurring salt that controlled a major psychiatric illness. It was hard to argue that it was covering up the cause of the illness. The biogenic amine hypothesis made depression more understandable and similar to other medical illnesses like thyroid disease, hypertension, or diabetes. Psychiatrists began to shift their treatment models from fifty-minute hours on couches or in plush offices to briefer appointments in examination rooms where patients were weighed and their blood pressures checked. There has been a slight shift back toward psychology in recent years. The current thinking is that patients who have both counseling and medication do better than either alone. There is some PET scan evidence that both therapeutic approaches affect the brain but in different areas, which makes the combination of the two more effective.

Mnemonics are memory helpers. **ROY G BIV** is a way to remember the colors of the rainbow (red, orange, yellow, green, blue, indigo, and violet). The two for depression are **SIG E CAPS** and **C GASP DIE.**

S=Suicidal thoughts
I=Interests decreased
G=Guilt
E=Energy decreased
C=Concentration decreased
A=Appetite disturbance
P=Psychomotor changes
S=Sleep disturbance

C=Concentration decreased
G=Guilt
A=Appetite disturbance
S=Sleep disturbance
P=Psychomotor retardation (or agitation)
D=Death or suicidal thoughts
I=Interests decreased
E=Energy decreased

This disorder typically responds to a combination of antidepressant medication and cognitive-behavioral therapy. A good place to start would, again, be your family physician. Tell your warrior you made an appointment for him and you will be going with him to the doctors to talk about something for sleep and something to help his appetite, energy level, libido, gastrointestinal complaints, etc. Call the nurse and tell her you think he is depressed. Let her know he is eligible for help from the VA. Let her know if you think he is at risk for self-harm.

Bipolar Depression

There is a type of depression that also runs in families that is characterized by periods of depression interspersed with periods of hyperactivity, hyperirritability, pressured thought, pressured speech, insomnia, sometimes hypersexuality, impulsivity, and impaired judgment. In the old days it was referred to as "folie circulaire" and later "manic depression." This form of depression occurs less frequently than the type of depression above, but it is necessary to recognize and diagnose because this form of depression does not respond as well to antidepressant medication (sometimes antidepressants can push a depressed bipolar patient into a manic episode) and the risk of suicide is generally higher in this type of depressive illness. Mood stabilizers and antipsychotics are the treatment of choice for most cases of bipolar affective illness. Lithium, Tegretol, Depakote, and Lamictal are the mood stabilizers that are commonly prescribed. Among antipsychotics, the newer atypical antipsychotics are more frequently used to treat this disorder.

It is important to ask warriors, regardless of which type of depression they are experiencing, if they are thinking of suicide. Family members and even professional caregivers are reluctant to ask about suicide because they don't want to put the idea in depressed people's heads and, even more common, they are afraid the individuals will say they are thinking of ending their life and they don't know what to do next. You may approach this topic by asking, "Do you feel hopeless and helpless at times?" If they admit they are, then ask, "Do you feel like giving up?" If they say yes then you can ask, "Do you ever think of ending it all?" If they admit they do, you can ask if they have specific plans to take their own life, how would they do it, do they have the means to do it, do they have plans as to what they want to happen after they die, etc.

Suicide

The escalating number of suicides among soldiers and veterans has captured the media's attention recently. Eighteen soldiers and veterans take their own lives daily, and this does not include those who die from risky behavior on motorcycles, automobiles, and other possible self-destructive activities. Suicide rates among veterans are approximately three times that of the general population. Suicide rates among individuals in the VA's care may be as high as 7.5 times the national average. One thousand suicide attempts per month occur among veterans seen in VA medical facilities. A recent study by the military notes multiple factors may be involved. Young soldiers have frequent moves, family problems, financial problems, exposure to danger, and in some cases exposure to death and injury of comrades. Also, 14 percent use opiate pain medicines, and one-third take a prescription drug. In their twenties they have the equivalent amount of stress as an eighty-year-old civilian has tolerated over a lifetime. There is also a stigma associated with getting mental health assistance, a lack of command awareness and empathy, and inability to admit weakness. Seventy-percent of those who took their own lives had no or only one deployment. This may suggest that those who have multiple deployments have more resiliency or some other factors are involved.

As noted in chapter one, General Patton set a macho tone for the military in World War II that equated battle fatigue with personal weakness and malingering. He called for soldiers to ridicule individuals who complained of these symptoms. As we noted, honor is important to soldiers, and appearing cowardly and weak in the presence of comrades in arms is probably the worst thing a warrior could imagine. It is important that the military overcome this image from the past and that men are convinced that brave men can ask for help without dishonor. Men tend to want to solve their own problems, and if they are backed into a corner, that solution may involve taking themselves out of the picture. Fortunately, the current military command, in an effort to stem the tide of suicides, has initiated a campaign to emphasize that it takes strength and courage to admit weaknesses and to seek help.

One of my psychiatric patients told me about her thirty-one-year-old nephew, who was a reservist. He was single and a college graduate. He had served two tours in Iraq and had considerable time "outside of the wire" in combat. He had witnessed close friends being killed and some who were wounded by IED explosions. He didn't have any mental health treatment himself, but his aunt (my patient) thought he should have. He was home a relatively short time when he received orders for a third tour, this time in Afghanistan. He was upset about receiving the orders. He seemed agitated but also withdrew from the family. He left a note for his parents telling them they would be better off without him. The family felt he had been upset by the terrible injuries his friends experienced from improvised explosive devices and was afraid he might experience the same. She said he was angry with himself for being afraid. His death was upsetting to my patient and for the rest of the family. They all said they wished he had received professional assistance for what appeared to them to be a depressive illness and irrational thinking on his part. They felt guilty for not taking steps to see that he saw a mental health professional.

Risk Factors for Suicide

- Young
- White
- Male
- National Guard or reservist
- Financial problems
- Family problems
- Chemical dependency
- Use of pain or prescription medications
- High stress level
- Zero to one deployments
- Lack of mental health attention or support
- History of previous attempts
- Family history of suicide or violence
- Talk about suicide
- Giving away possessions
- Talk about plans after death

- Writing instructions in the event of death
- No future plans
- Suddenly visiting old friends and family members
- Sudden change in mood or behavior
- Risk-taking behaviors
- Agitation or violent behavior
- Chemical dependency
- Stopping or changing medications
- To progress in treatment for a while
- Presence of physical illness or injury
- A major loss
- A significant life change
- Feeling alone
- Other friends, relatives, or acquaintances committing suicide

As noted earlier, caregivers, including some professionals, are frequently reluctant to ask if people are thinking of suicide. They worry about putting ideas in their heads and also are afraid if they say "yes" they won't know what to do next. When I am interviewing patients on this topic, I start out with a general question: "Do you ever feel like giving up?" If they say they do, then I ask, "Do you ever think of suicide?" If they answer in the affirmative, I ask, "Have you thought how you would do it?" I then inquire to see if they have thought out how they might take their lives and if they have the means to do it. For example, if they say they've thought of shooting themselves and that they have access to a loaded weapon, that is pretty specific and dangerous. I would then ask that their relative remove anything handy that they might use to hurt themselves. This is important because most suicides are impulsive, and if items that could be used to take the person's life are not immediately available, the risk is greatly reduced in many cases. For example, in England a few years ago the suicide rates dropped dramatically. At first professionals thought this was due to improved educational and preventive programs. They were surprised to learn that the decreased mortality was due to the gas companies switching from coke gas to a less toxic cooking gas in homes. Sticking one's head into an oven was a popular means of suicide in England, and when the ability to impulsively end one's life in that manner was eliminated, the death rate dropped.

Having determined that a person is thinking of suicide and having eliminated the immediate access to a means of self-harm, I continue to ask about future plans. Does the person have plans for what to do with his or her possessions after death? Is the patient giving away things? Has the person made an effort to visit friends or family members and say good-bye? Did the patient get insurance papers or a will in order? In other words, is the person preparing for death? This is a much more dangerous situation. On the other hand, if the person is planning to go to college next year or take the kids on vacation, his or her future plans seem to be to alive, and this lessens the risk.

Another factor that greatly increases the danger of suicide is alcohol. One-third of all suicides are committed by men addicted to alcohol, and chemical dependency increases the risk for suicide five times in a depressed man. Under the influence the individual's judgment is suspended, his impulsivity is increased, and he is likely to be more depressed.

If you decide your warrior is thinking toward the future, has no immediate means to harm him- or herself, and is just having fleeting thoughts of suicide that the person is not likely to act upon, you could then inquire what the soldier could do when those thoughts arise. If your loved one doesn't come up with it, you could suggest that he or she let you know when those thoughts arrive.

Of course, if a person has even fleeting thoughts of suicide it means the depression is serious and professional assistance is needed. In most cases this means seeing a psychiatrist. If you feel the person is in immediate danger of self-harm, you may need to enlist the help of a crisis team or the police to physically restrain him and convey him to the nearest emergency room for evaluation and probable hospitalization.

Panic Disorder

The mnemonic to remember the symptoms of panic disorder is **STUDENTS FEAR the 3 Cs.**

S=Sweating
T=Trembling
U=Unsteadiness/dizziness
D=Derealization/depersonalization
E=Elevated heart rate (tachycardia)
N=Nausea
T=Tingling
S=Shortness of breath
F=Fear of dying

F=Fear of losing control
F=Fear of going crazy
C=Choking
C=Chest pain
C=Chills

Panic disorder is a common condition that affects one-third of young adults have at least one and 2 percent of people worldwide develop a panic disorder. It occurs in 25 percent of close relatives, and there appears to be a genetic component to the illness. It is frequently seen associated with both depression and PTSD. Victims of panic disorder feel that they are hypochondriacs, but there is a physical basis for the illness. If you give a person who is predisposed to panic disorder intravenous sodium lactate, you can precipitate an attack.

One theory as to the origin of panic disorder is it is a primitive protective mechanism that we no longer need. If a baby lion is separated from its mother in the jungle, as soon as it realizes it is alone it freezes. It doesn't move or make a sound. The mother sniffs around and locates it. The catatonic state keeps it from being discovered by predators. It is thought that humans have a similar mechanism that is more prominent genetically in some families. The person gets in a situation where he or she has no control, has a panic attack, and then the attacks continue. They may be brought on by anything that reminds the person of the initial (herald) attack.

Patients report they feel as though they are going to die or go crazy when they have one of these attacks. They often avoid anything they associate with the attack. For example, if a person has one in a doctor's waiting room, then going to the doctor, being in a crowded room, smelling alcohol or odors that were in the physician's office, or feeling sick can precipitate another attack. In addition, the symptoms of the disorder itself (rapid breathing, light-headedness, rapid heartbeat, dizziness, etc.) can bring on an attack as well. Typically patients think they are having a heart attack or a seizure and usually have multiple physical workups prior to getting to the psychiatrist for help. We used to have a support group in our office that consisted of individuals with panic disorder who were recovering. Most had been isolated by their illness, and they enjoyed interacting with others who shared many common experiences. One of the group members was a musician who brought his guitar to a meeting and sang a song he had composed called "I'm a Hypochondriac." Among the lyrics: "Gee, I think I'm having a heart attack, and oh my aching back." His final stanza was, "But my doctors really like me, and they even like my ills, because I'm a hypochondriac who pays his medical bills."

In the old days in nearly every small town there would be at least one recluse who remained isolated in his or her home. Usually this was an individual who suffered from panic attacks and had retreated until remaining at home, often with a relative who looked after the recluse because, in addition to be afraid of going out, the person was afraid of being alone as well. We used to say a recluse had "neurasthenia" or a "weak heart."

When I started practice, the treatment for panic disorder was to refer the patient to a therapist who would ask the person to list the ten things he or she most feared. Then the counselor would have the patient visualize each one and then relax. After the patient was able to get through the list of ten and stay relaxed, the therapist would have the patient actually go out and face them (go to the mall, go out to dinner, cross a bridge, etc.). We prescribed minor tranquilizers, and we had a support group to cheer the patient on. We used these methods to treat panic disorder for a number of years. Then a psychiatrist in England wrote a paper on the successful treatment of panic disorder using monomine oxidase inhibitors. This was a surprise for US psychiatrists, who reserved these drugs (Nardil, Parnate, Marplan) for treatment-resistant depression. These potent drugs had many side effects and interacted with many other drugs. When the drugs were first used in Italy, several patients had strokes and it was found that they were eating aged cheese and drinking Chianti red wine. Chemical analysis showed these two foods were high in tyramine and that tyramine and an MAOI could cause a release of epinephrine in the body followed by a sudden spike in blood pressure. Patients on MAOIs are required to follow a tyramine-free diet. I pulled the charts on all of our patients with panic disorder, told them about the paper, and asked them if they wanted to try the MAOI. They all did, so they weren't satisfied with what we had been doing. We put them on Nardil, and they all got better. Of course these were apprehensive patients, and the first question they had when we said we had a drug that would help them was, "What's it going to do to me?" When we said that death due to stroke was one of the potential side effects, their anxiety was not lessened. We put together a support group of patients who were on Nardil. New patients wouldn't believe us but did believe people who were actually taking the medicine. We'd line each new patient up with a veteran who was taking the drug as his or her "prayer buddy." The new patient would go home, take the pill, sit on the bed, and start feeling funny. The patient would look at the can of peas he or she had for dinner and, sure enough, it would contain MSG. The person would suspect a reaction to the Nardil. The new patient would then call the "prayer buddy," who would reassure him or her that it was a panic attack and not a reaction and that it took four to six weeks to get results and to hang in there and the person would be fine. We went on using Nardil for several years until the American Psychiatric Association asked three top psychopharmacologists to write a protocol for the treatment of panic disorder. They asked, "Do you want us to write what is in the literature or what we are doing?" "What's the difference?" they were asked.

"Well, in the literature the treatment is Nardil, Imipramine, and Xanax," they answered. "But we are using SSRIs and they are effective." Once this word got out, all the psychiatrists switched to SSRIs because they didn't require special precautions and they didn't react adversely with many medications. This is the treatment of panic disorder today: an SSRI (Prozac, Zoloft, Paxil, Luvox, Celexa, Lexapro, etc.) and Xanax for the anticipatory anxiety. Patients often inquire if they should push themselves to do things, and I tell them no because they want to do things and, as soon as the medicine starts to alleviate the panic attacks, they will go ahead and do all of the things they were avoiding because they will know that they are over the scary episodes.

For warriors, panic attacks are extra stressful because they feel like wimps not being able to get out and do the things they want to do. I once saw a Special Forces sergeant who said that he was decorated for sitting in the front of his vehicle manning a gun when, because of his seniority, he could have been riding in the enclosed rear. He said, "Heck, Doc, I've got panic attacks—I couldn't stand to be closed up in the back of that vehicle!" In civilian practice I once saw a high school buddy of mine named Ted for an emergency appointment on a Saturday morning. This fellow was a big, husky football star in high school who ran a hot air balloon business on the West Coast. He took part in daring activities—skydiving, scuba diving, and snowboarding—and he was definitely a "macho man." Ted was flying across the country and had to change planes in O'Hare Airport in Chicago. He had a panic attack in the airport and had to call his mother in Bloomington, Indiana, to come get him. The following day I saw him in my office, where he sat frustrated and angry with himself. "Can you imagine, I had to have my mother come and get me!" he exclaimed. He said, "I've got to be the biggest chicken shit guy you've ever seen." I reassured him that panic disorder was a common, genetically determined chemical abnormality that was treatable and did not reflect on his manhood or ability to control himself. He responded to an SSRI and returned to his usual risky activities without limitation.

Some patients with anxiety and panic disorder discover that alcohol dampens these symptoms. In some cases this leads to an additional problem of addiction. Those with panic disorder also find that "the morning after" is a time when they are likely to experience an attack. Their alcohol blood level drops and they become shaky, often precipitating a panic attack.

Chemical Dependency

According to the National Survey on Drug Use and Health Report, one-quarter of veterans twenty-five and under suffer from substance abuse disorders. Chemical dependency remains one of the top three diagnoses in the VA system.

Is the warrior addicted? If you are concerned, he or she probably is. Here are the criteria used by the National Institute on Alcohol Abuse and Alcoholism to determine if someone is addicted:

- A man should have no more than four drinks a day and no more than fourteen a week.

- Does he put himself at risk while drinking? Does he drink and drive?

- Has drinking caused problems in his relationships?

- Has it caused problems at work, academically, or with the family?

- Are there legal problems related to drinking?

- Has he been unable to stop?

- Has he been unable to limit his drinking?

- Has he developed a tolerance to alcohol, requiring more of it to achieve the same effects?

- Has he shown signs of withdrawal, such as tremors, sweating, nausea, irritability, and insomnia when not drinking?

- Has he continued to drink despite having problems as a result of drinking?

- Is he spending lots of time drinking, thinking about drinking, or recovering from drinking?

- Has he spent less time on other matters because of drinking?

Men have difficulty recognizing their feelings. They know they feel bad, but they have a difficult time identifying depression or anxiety. Typically they will try to solve their unhappiness through self-medication or other compulsive activity. Most frequently this involves alcohol or drugs or both. In Vietnam alcohol and drugs were plentiful and cheap. Officers and senior NCOs drank while enlisted men used drugs. In OIF and OEF drugs and alcohol are less accessible in most cases. However, the use of prescription drugs has doubled, and 14 percent of the troops are taking some sort of pain medication.

While we typically think of a male when we think of an alcoholic, women become addicted to alcohol more rapidly. It may take longer to recognize that a woman is addicted and longer for her to "hit bottom" and see the need for abstinence and treatment.

Mnemonics for substance addiction are **ADDICTeD** and **WILD**:

A=Activities are given up or reduced
D=Dependence, physical tolerance
D=Dependency, physical withdrawal
I=Interpersonal (internal) consequences, physical or psychological
C=Can't cut down or control use
T=Time-consuming
D=Duration or amount of use is greater than intended

W=Work, school, or home role obligation failures
I=Interpersonal or social consequences
L=Legal problems
D=Dangerous use

Alcohol does dampen anxiety. It also relieves guilt temporarily. The Freudians used to say that the superego (conscience) was the alcohol-soluble portion of the personality. The problem is that when the individual becomes dependent on it, he now has two problems. Some patients come to me and want me to treat their anxiety and depressive symptoms, and then they will give up alcohol. I tell them that this won't work. They must first stop using, and then we'll try to work on the depression and anxiety. Patients never say they are addicted and this is why they need a drug or alcohol. Instead they say they need to sleep or they can't stand their anxiety. In the same way, patients don't say they are addicted to pain medicine. Instead, they say they are having severe pain and need relief.

Coercion Is Frequently Necessary and Often Effective

When I was in charge of the inpatient psychiatric unit at Ireland Army Hospital at Fort Knox in 1969, I developed an alcohol treatment program. Those having alcohol-related problems in their unit, who repeatedly came to the emergency room with alcohol-related problems, who had domestic violence or child abuse problems that were alcohol related, or had a DUI on post were referred to my program, and their spouses and commanding officers were notified. My program consisted of daily attendance at AA, group therapy three days a week, and Antabuse given daily by the spouse. The Antabuse made individuals deathly ill if they attempted to drink while it was in their system. It also reassured the spouses who gave it to them daily that they were not drinking. If an individual failed to attend an AA or group therapy meeting, or to take his daily Antabuse, the spouse, the commanding officer, and I were notified. If this pattern of noncompliance continued, the individual would be discharged from the military as a general 212 administrative discharge. New members of my program complained, "You said this was a voluntary program—it isn't voluntary!" "It's sort of voluntary," I would reply. Later, a number of men thanked me for forcing them to do what they knew they should do. When I left for Vietnam, we had several men who were doing well with their sobriety. The point of this is that coercion is frequently necessary, and it is often effective in getting the addict the help he or she needs. Addicts are afraid of giving up their "best friend" (the drug of choice). For all of us, change is frightening because it is the unknown. In addition, the initial abstinence from alcohol is likely to be accompanied by withdrawal symptoms characterized by restlessness, irritability, and discontented feelings (RID). We used to say that until people hit bottom, they won't be willing to try to stop their addiction. In other words, unless the anxiety, pain, or depression associated with continuing the addiction is not greater than that of abstaining and drying out, the person is unlikely to stop. Threatened divorce by the wife, threatened loss of gainful employment, threatened death from liver failure, threatened loss of love from the children—any of these may be enough to motivate the individual to seek treatment. Considerable external pressure is often necessary to initially force the individual into treatment.

Some treatment programs have a rigid structure, and patients who don't accept their particular approach are seen as unmotivated and are rejected. AA is a twelve-step, self-help program, and recovery is felt to be dependent on accepting and following the steps that are outlined in the big book. AA says that rehabilitation services are $60,000 treatment programs that tell addicts to go to AA. Other programs accept a wide range of treatment modalities in order to attempt to include a wide variety of addicted individuals. Peter Novotny was a Viennese psychoanalyst at the Menninger Clinic who supervised me during my residency training. He said, "When dealing with addiction, it is wise not to be too hard or too soft." What he meant was if the caregiver was too hard and demanded immediate sobriety and absolute compliance to treatment, he frequently lost the patient, who quit and went elsewhere. On the other hand, if the professional was too soft and acquiesced to all of the patient's demands, the patient would remain addicted and never recover. For example, I had an alcoholic patient years ago who would come to see me for his panic attacks. He was unable to stop drinking, and I encouraged him to go into rehabilitation for detoxification. He always had a reason why that particular time was not the right time. He had things to do at work. His children were having a celebration. Someone in the family was ill. He did start to sign up on a couple of occasions but then would back out at the last moment. I continued to follow him for four years while he continued to drink and refuse my recommendations. Finally, after four years, he went along with my suggestions and went into the hospital to detoxify and take part in the rehabilitation program. He has been sober and active in AA for nearly twenty years now. I think of him as a patient who was successfully treated by following Dr. Novotny's approach.

Drugs

It has been estimated that a quarter of the soldiers twenty-five and under have a problem with drugs. There is a 25 percent increase in returning veterans seeking help for substance abuse problems. The number of prescriptions for pain medicines among troops has doubled, and 14 percent of returning troops are taking an opiate pain medication of some type (95 percent Oxycontin). As Command Sergeant Major Huber notes, many of the troops carry one hundred pounds of equipment and develop muscular and joint trauma and pain. Many take "vitamin M" (Motrin), and a number become dependent on pain medicines to relieve their chronic aches and pains. Twenty-eight thousand troops were discharged in a year for misconduct. Some critics allege that a good share of these soldiers were suffering from mental health and substance abuse problems.

VIII. Ideas for the Future

"*The willingness with which our young people are likely to serve in any war, no matter how justified, shall be directly proportional as to how they perceive veterans of earlier wars and how they were treated and appreciated by this country.*"

— George Washington

President Kennedy quoted the following verse in 1962 to the men of the Army's First Armored Division who had been moved into position during the Cuban missile crisis:

God and the soldier, all men adore

In time of danger and not before.

When the danger is passed and all things righted,

God is forgotten, and the soldier slighted.

It is important that we remember our veterans and their families as we withdraw from Iraq and Afghanistan. In this time of economic crises, we may be tempted to neglect their needs. This would be morally wrong and a threat to our future security should we make this mistake.

I'm not a military expert, but in my opinion, we need to go slow when it comes to cutting funds for the military. Our nation's security is at stake. We've concluded recently that future wars will be against terrorists and that we need small, highly trained Special Forces to deal with this type of conflict. Again, I'm just a layperson, but it would seem to me that any conflict with Russia or China is likely to involve large-scale, more conventional warfare, and we should prepare for this possibility as well.

The best minds in the military and mental health fields are struggling with ideas to meet the future mental health needs of our veterans and their families. We've seen the statistics that demonstrate an increasing incidence of PTSD, TBIs, mTBIs, depression, chemical dependency, divorce, child abuse, financial difficulties, unemployment, incarceration, and homelessness among veterans and their families. The military is short staffed and having difficulty recruiting and retaining sufficient numbers of mental health professionals. In addition, the quality of those being recruited has been questioned. The resources to deal with these needs are limited due to the current national economic crisis.

It has been found that over twenty-eight thousand soldiers were kicked out of the army since the war in Iraq started on the basis of personality disorder and misconduct. Their records showed that, after their return from OEF or OIF, they were diagnosed with PTSD or other mental health disorders. They subsequently broke army rules, sometimes the law, and some began using illegal drugs. These behaviors led to less than honorable discharges. As a result, they were denied medical and other military benefits, although seemingly the misbehavior was a product of their mental difficulties. Psychiatrist Jonathan Shay wondered why they were accepted by the military if they had personality disorders and if the use of this stigmatizing diagnosis might not be a way of avoiding paying these veterans disability compensation.

VIII. Ideas for the Future

This chapter contains my ideas and suggestions as to how we might attempt to address these concerns despite our monetary shortfalls.

Decreasing the Number of Deployments

Since the all-volunteer military was instituted in 1973, the demand for soldiers to deploy for combat overseas (most recently OIF and OEF) has increased while the number of troops serving has decreased. This has resulted in multiple deployments. Sergeant First Class Ronald A. Grider was killed Tuesday, September 28, 2010, at 9:47 p.m. during his ninth deployment. Jeff Hanks, married with two small daughters and an infantryman with the 101st who had two previous deployments, to Iraq and Afghanistan, went AWOL rather than board a plane to Kuwait and his third deployment back to Afghanistan. He was diagnosed with PTSD by two civilian psychiatrists and was being evaluated at Fort Campbell when his command made him leave for his third hardship tour. A nephew of one of my patients committed suicide after receiving his orders for his third deployment.

It seems if something isn't done to alleviate the problems of multiple deployments, there will be little hope to reduce the increasing rates of mental problems and family problems in the military. The military organization is going to have greater difficulty recruiting new troops and retaining old troops unless this situation is corrected. Another effect of the volunteer army is the need for the military to pay attention to the needs and wishes of the troops' spouses and children. If they are unhappy, it is unlikely that the soldier will reenlist, and if they do not feel welcome, it is doubtful that they will support enlistment in the first place. While high unemployment rates and a poor economy may cause many to consider military service, recruitment and retention depend, in large part, on the goodwill of spouses and families. In addition, marital and family stresses appear to be significant factors in the suicides and postdeployment mental problems of many soldiers. Greater emphasis could be placed on helping soldiers think through their decision to marry and the spouses they have chosen. We know that the couples are often young and lack knowledge and preparation for marriage. Marriage enrichment courses specifically designed to help military newlyweds communicate, share financial decisions, learn to parent, and develop a deep, committed relationship could be developed. Help from chaplains, ministers, and more mature military personnel who enjoy good, trusting relationships could be utilized in this regard. Newlyweds could be encouraged to socialize with other happily married military couples who could monitor them and serve as marriage sponsors. Programs like BATTLEMIND, resiliency programs training, and the efforts to recruit more mental health professionals are small steps in the direction of trying to cope with the increasing rates of mental health problems, suicides, family problems, TBI, and chemical dependency among returning troops. However, it is unlikely that these efforts will be successful unless something is done to reduce the number of redeployments. This essentially means that either the need for combat troops is reduced worldwide or the number of combat troops is increased. We are pulling out of Iraq and talking about getting out of Afghanistan, so possibly the demand for warriors will be lessened. If the number of deployments can be decreased, stress to the troops and their families will be decreased. Fewer deployments may make it easier to recruit and retain troops in the future. Another solution that has been proposed would be to reinstitute the draft. Perhaps this could be two years of obligatory service for men and women after high school, with options to serve in public service or the military. This should be a national draft that would be fair to everyone. However it is accomplished, redeployment is a key factor leading to the high rates of mental health and family problems. Something must be done to reduce the number of combat tours if these statistics are going to be improved.

VIII. Ideas for the Future

"Dwell time" (the time home between deployments) has been shown to be important to soldiers' mental health. Mental health problems in maneuver units returned to near garrison rates (about 10 percent with problems) after twenty-four months of dwell time and completely returned after thirty to thirty-six months.

Physical training during off time was associated with a reduction in mental health problems, as was no more than three or four hours of Internet surfing and video games.

Reducing the Stigma of Asking for Help for Mental Problems

The heritage of General Patton has not yet faded away. As we've seen, both warriors and their spouses are reluctant to seek help because of the fear that it will harm their chances for promotion. A study of deployed soldiers who were screened for TBI and mTBI noted that a significant number cheated on the examination so they would not be sent home and leave their buddies in the field. The military has an active advertising campaign in place that indicates it takes courage to ask for help. One of the army's twelve four-star generals, Carter Ham, has spoken openly of his own PTSD, which may be an important influence in changing the military's attitude toward receiving professional help for psychiatric problems. The military respects and identifies with its leaders. If the top brass say something is OK, everyone below them will as well. When I was in Vietnam, the commanding general and his staff had short World War II-style burr haircuts and were clean-shaven. Although there were no orders about officer grooming, all of the career military officers in the division followed suit.

In the First Infantry Division in 1969, a psychotic soldier went into a bunker, shot and killed six soldiers, and then turned the gun on himself. Investigation revealed he had been behaving bizarrely for some time prior to the tragic event. His commanding officer

(CO) felt it was his responsibility to solve his men's problems and had not referred him to me, the division psychiatrist, or even to the unit's battalion surgeon or chaplain. The commanding general asked me to write a paper on the warning signs of mental illness to be distributed to COs in the division, with the admonishment that division commanders were to send any soldiers who appeared to be having problems to the division psychiatrist. Referrals escalated after this. In other words, what the top brass says and does has a powerful influence on the behavior of the organization.

Another excellent suggestion to help returning veterans get the mental health assistance they need was offered recently by a waiting wife. She noted that civilian policemen who shoot someone while on duty are required to see a therapist for a prescribed number of visits. They are assumed to have been traumatized by the experience. Soldiers who shoot someone while serving in a combat area, on the other hand, are expected to cope with this event on their own. She said she wished all returning combat veterans, like civilian police officers, were required to see a therapist for a number of visits. She said this would bypass the warrior's resistance to asking for psychological help as well as much of the stigma associated with mental health treatment in the military. To meet the additional needs for counselors to accomplish this task, combat veterans who successfully made the postdeployment adjustment to civilian life could be trained as counselors to provide these services.

As we described earlier, the online cognitive-behavioral program to treat PTSD and other programs like the one for stress reduction that is used by the chaplains corps are fairly inexpensive, easily accessible, confidential, and effective approaches that could be utilized by large numbers of individuals. These approaches do not require the recruitment of mental health caregivers by the military or the VA.

VIII. Ideas for the Future

Normal Reactions to Abnormal Situations

I agree with Colonel Hoge, author of *Once a Warrior—Always a Warrior*, that the problems of PTSD are largely due to the persistence of behaviors from combat into civilian life. In this book we've traced their development in basic and advanced individual training to that of the combat zone itself. If we understand the symptoms of PTSD in this light as the natural carryover of behaviors developed to survive and respond to stress in combat, they will seem less mysterious and frightening than some sort of mental illness that developed due to war. The undoing of these symptoms may also appear to be more possible and logical to veterans and families. At the same time, we've learned recently from PET scans that PTSD causes physical changes in the structure and functioning of the brain. It is a physical illness just like TBI and mTBI. However, as my military counseling friends remind me, patterns carried over from a dysfunctional, trauma-ridden childhood can predispose individuals to problems in the military and in combat—including PTSD. In other words, a person who grew up being traumatized as a child may not require as much combat trauma to develop symptoms of PTSD. Also, the combat trauma need not be one horrendous event—it may be the daily threat of danger. It is important to take a complete psychosocial history and include these factors when evaluating a veteran who is symptomatic. Education of the returning soldier and his or her family is useful. If the veteran and the family can understand the etiology of the returning warrior's symptoms as well as the treatment to alleviate the symptoms, the problem becomes less frightening.

The military has developed BATTLEMIND training programs for soldiers and families and more recently instituted resiliency training for both. It raises the awareness of the soldiers and their families of the behaviors that are necessary in combat that later become troubling during civilian life and offers suggestions to lessen the stresses and ease readjustment. This program recognizes that both veterans and their families have unrealistic expectations of their reunions after deployment. Suggestions are made for both the warriors and those at home about how they can lower their expectations and prepare for a more realistic adjustment period. The military is enthusiastic about resiliency training as a cure-all for its obvious mental health problems. It reminds me of our local hospital administration having all of its professional staff members go through Steven Covey's *7 Habits of Highly Effective People* training, hoping that this would relieve their organizational difficulties. The hospital administration was impressed by Covey's book and thought it was the answer to all of the administrative shortcomings. Unfortunately it proved not to be the case. Far from a final answer to the current problems, resiliency training probably ably represents, as the movie *What About Bob?* describes, "baby steps." They are steps in the right direction in terms of recognizing the need to focus attention on the mental health needs of the troops and their families, but obviously there is a long way to go to be able to make a difference in the mental health problems of soldiers and their loved ones. And again, if something isn't done to increase troop strength and decrease the number of deployments by each individual soldier, there is little hope that the mental and family problems will lessen.

It seems to me that the military could devote some money, time, and energy reversing the training it has invested in soldiers and warriors to "untrain" them prior to their returning to civilian life. This would not be in the context of psychotherapy but rather undoing some of the patterns that were instilled during military training. Group meetings with other veterans might include discussions on the morality of war and the justification for killing the enemy. Guilt from killing another human being (or supporting the killing of another individual) is a great stress for many combat veterans. It is also a topic that has been avoided by the military and many mental health professionals in the past. Survival guilt needs to be dealt with

VIII. Ideas for the Future

as well—what causes it, and what to do about the depression and guilt that many soldiers experience. An investment in educational programs, marriage enrichment programs, and mentoring for new recruits and their wives may help reduce the problems, divorces, child abuse, and probably some of the suicides that result from family difficulties in the military.

Reducing Unit Stress in the Combat Zone

The military has developed some uniform guidelines for its professional caregivers. This is new and a positive step. When I was in the service, we had a brief introduction to military psychiatry at Fort Sam Houston during our basic officer's training course. I was fortunate to be assigned to Fort Knox for a year before I deployed to Vietnam, and this gave me one year's practical experience with military psychiatry. I attempted to review the military psychiatry literature while at Fort Knox and in Vietnam. This self-education helped as well. Sergeant De Leon was the psychiatric ward master on my unit at Ireland Army Hospital. He shared his twenty-year experience working on psychiatry services, including that of working with Dr. Roy Grinker in World War II. We conducted some sodium amytal interviews based on his tutelage. My preparation for the job of the First Infantry Division's psychiatrist consisted of a brief course at Fort Sam Houston, one year's experience in military psychiatry at Fort Knox, on-the-job training from the experienced ward master, and self-study of the military psychiatry literature. In comparison with most of my nonmilitary-trained peers, I was probably pretty well prepared to take the First Infantry Division psychiatry assignment. However, it would have been much better had I been given formal instruction for the job. By formal training I mean specifically classroom instruction on the history of military psychiatry and step-by-step instruction as to what a division psychiatrist's duties were in a combat zone and how to carry them out in the best possible manner. At the same time, it would have been helpful had men who were training to be commanding officers in a combat division were also instructed as to what they might expect from their division psychiatrists and mental health workers in the division and how best to utilize their services. No doubt graduates of this hypothetical program would have to adapt what they learned to the nuances of their combat assignments, but they would be better prepared to carry out their mission if they were formally trained in advance. Our division surgeon did have all new battalion surgeons coming to the division stop by our division psychiatry service so that we could brief them on what we were doing and what we could offer them in terms of psychiatric/mental health support. This provided personal contact with the docs and made it easier for them to contact us and refer soldiers from their units in the future.

Guidelines for professional mental health workers are positive "baby steps" for professional training. I am sure the services have included some of the lessons learned from Vietnam and subsequent conflicts in the curriculum of the professionals who train in the military. I was a board examiner for the American Board of Psychiatry and Neurology for a number of years. The team I served on was led by M. J. Martin, who was the chief of psychiatry at the Mayo Clinic and a colonel in the Army Reserve. As a result, he invited several senior military psychiatrists to serve on our team over the years, and a number of them said they used my papers from Vietnam as part of their curriculum for teaching military psychiatric residents. Currently, the military is urging its mental health workers in OIF and OEF to travel to the units to consult and to not stay in the base camps because of fear of IEDs. I think this is the right idea, but again it would be helpful to give more specific instructions on what to do when the professionals consult with line units. Which units should the psychiatric consultants see? How can stress in the units be identified? What is the format for a unit consultation? What data should be collected, and how should it be fed back to the unit?

VIII. Ideas for the Future

How can the effectiveness of the consultation be measured? These are some of the questions that might be answered in a structured program offered to mental health teams prior to their attempting to consult with line units. I wish that I had had classroom instruction on the history of military psychiatry, courses as to the duties and optimal functioning of a division psychiatrist, information about the typical problems mental health workers might see in a combat zone, etc. Also, information about backup services available to mental health personnel in the combat area would have been useful. Current technology would permit professionals in the field to consult with senior military psychiatrists in the States. These well-trained, experienced professionals could provide invaluable support to mental health workers in combat areas.

I did my psychiatric residency training at the Menninger School of Psychiatry in Topeka, Kansas. William Menninger had been a brigadier general and the head of army psychiatry during World War II. He started a section of industrial psychiatry at the Menninger Foundation that was later headed by Harry Levinson, PhD. I served on Dr. Levinson's faculty for his seminars for executive training in mental health. (Top executives of companies with fifty thousand employees or more were invited to participate in a weeklong intensive seminar on the mental health aspects of management in Topeka. A separate seminar was held for industrial physicians.) My senior paper was based on an organizational study of Topeka State Hospital under Dr. Levinson's supervision. Dr. Levinson has published a number of best-selling books in the business field and has served on the faculty of the Harvard School of Business. He applied individual assessment and psychodynamics to the evaluation and intervention with organizations. I attempted to apply his approach in a simplistic and crude manner to the First Infantry Division in Vietnam. At our division headquarters, we noted that we would periodically receive a number of referrals from the same unit, and rather than passing out Valium to several soldiers, we felt it would be more effective to go to the unit and see what was going on there that might be causing the stress that led to these referrals. We kept track of disciplinary rates (court-martials, 212s), malaria rates (because this was an indicator of unit discipline), chaplain referrals, psychiatric referrals, VD rates, etc., as "stress indicators" for each unit. We would graph these statistics, and when we saw a rise in several of the stress indicators for a particular unit we would visit the unit to identify the source of stress. We had the support of our division surgeon, who in turn was a close friend of the division's commanding general. With his help, we contacted the commanding officer of the particular unit we'd identified and met with him and his staff officers to explain what we'd observed and to offer our assistance to him. We reassured him that the process would be confidential and would not affect his record in any way. Our division surgeon helped by recommending us and our work to the commanding officer in advance. With the CO's approval, we then interviewed members of his chain of command as well as enlisted men in the unit. In some cases, one of our technicians stayed with the unit for a period to observe the unit from within and to gather additional information for our consultation.

An example of our unit intervention was a unit where an attempted assassination of a new commander occurred. We observed that change of command was often stressful for units. The men had come to trust their lives to the judgment of a particular commander, and when he became short, there was apprehension about the new CO who was about to assume command. This anxiety was greater because the departing CO let down his guard and tried to be friends with his men before he left. Rumors in the unit about the new commander were rife. A grenade was detonated in his hootch the evening of his arrival. We determined that, psychologically, the unit was angry at the departing CO but couldn't recognize this fact. After all, he was popular and he was entitled to leave after he put in his yearlong tour. The negative feelings were transferred to the

VIII. Ideas for the Future

new officer, whom no one knew and who hadn't even arrived in the unit. They reached a peak when someone set off the grenade. We interviewed the officers and men of the unit and prepared a lengthy report of our observations and suggestions and then fed the information in the report back to the unit, starting with the commanding officer. We discussed the need for the departing CO to tighten up his unit before he left and be stricter with his discipline, which would permit the men to express some of their negative feelings directly toward him. I told them that this was a common phenomenon. We passed on our findings to the other units in the division with the suggestion that departing COs be aware of these negative feelings and how by directing them to themselves they would be making the job easier for their predecessors. I can think of an example in private practice of a physician whose popular partner died and he took over his cases. No matter what he did, the patients were angry with him. He came to me because he was depressed about the death of his friend and partner and was upset about his inability to please his partner's patients. I pointed out that they weren't angry with him; they were angry with his partner for leaving them but couldn't express these feelings because their physician had died and it obviously wasn't his choice or his fault. A new minister in our church found a chilly reception while trying to replace a popular minister who retired. Despite his best efforts, nothing he did seemed to be right initially.

In retrospect, discussing the dynamics of stress in the unit, paying attention to the unit, and mirroring the members' own comments to them all seemed to have a positive effect in terms of reducing stress. I felt much of this was probably an example of the "Hawthorne effect," which occurred in a research project at the Western Electric Company in Chicago. In this study, an effort was made to determine the relationship between the intensity of light and a worker's productivity. Lighting was adjusted to different levels in different areas of the plant, and workers were interviewed before and after the adjustments were made. To the researchers' surprise, all areas of the plant showed increased productivity. The conclusion was that talking to workers increases productivity.

In our work with unit consultation in the First Infantry Division, the data we fed back to the units appeared to be helpful in most cases. Paying attention to the unit's ideas and concerns probably had a positive effect as well. Stress indices went down after our unit interventions in nearly all cases. I think this approach may have merit for today's military, especially utilizing current technology to monitor stress levels experienced by each unit. Stress monitoring and the consultation methods themselves could be much more sophisticated and effective utilizing modern technology. Mental health teams today are encouraged to consult with units, but it isn't clear what is involved in the consultation or how the intervention is to be carried out. Do the mental health workers wear the same unit patches as the units to which they consult? What rank do the consultants hold? It would be helpful if step-by-step instruction could be provided for these teams to tell them how to carry out a unit consultation and intervention. It would also be useful to set up some type of monitoring system to identify units that were experiencing stress and to follow these indicators after unit intervention by the mental health team was completed. Another significant point is the rank of the mental health professionals carrying out the consultation. I was a major in Vietnam, which permitted me to talk with some of the senior officers, but I would have been more effective had I been of higher rank. Also, my military experience was limited. Had I had more years in service, especially in combat areas, I would have enjoyed more respect and easier access to the unit cadre. In my particular case, my division surgeon, who was held in high esteem by the commanding general of the division, intervened and made up for some of my shortcomings by introducing me to the commanding officers and reassuring them that I was OK and could be useful to them. In Vietnam we noted that

VIII. Ideas for the Future

racial conflict appeared to be a major problem for many units. I was inexperienced and had no training in dealing with these difficulties. A senior officer of a different ethnic background would have been more effective in this regard. It would be of value to assign senior mental health professionals as consultants in the field. They would have direct access to senior commanders in the units and would be better able to effectively consult with them. It might also be possible to train senior NCOs with combat experience to consult with NCOs in the field on issues related to mental health. Our techs were enlisted men who wore the same patch as the men they served. Soldier/patients found it easier to confide in them because they were enlisted men and members of their division. Finally, I know the military uses visual communication. It would be possible to set up visual (and e-mail) links for psychiatrists in the combat area with senior psychiatrists at home who could serve as mentors to help them with difficult problems and advise them in their day-to-day duties in the field. I believe that most former combat psychiatrists who have left the military would be happy to pass on their experience and wisdom to new men in the field if they could do so in a convenient manner. (Few would want to end up like Dr. John Wicks, who was sent to Iraq to serve at age 68.) In a very rudimentary manner we were breaking new ground with our consultation efforts in Vietnam. I wish that I had been given formal instruction prior to my service there. I hope that present and future psychiatrists and mental health workers will have course work that will inform them about approaches that seemed promising in the past and provide them with structure for their work in the field. It would seem to me that they could benefit from day-to-day mentoring from senior military psychiatrists. Backup chemical dependency services and the ability to call in senior consultants to work with unit commanders might be helpful as well. War is the father of invention. The military offers an opportunity to research techniques of prevention in psychiatry that are not readily available in the civilian community.

KP and Exercise Programs to Reduce Problems

Roman soldiers were assigned to build aqueducts and other civic projects when they were standing down from combat in the field. Roman commanders knew that leaving them idle was asking for problems. My good friend, Vietnam veteran, and experienced soldier Command Sergeant Gary Huber suggests a regular program of physical exercise for deployed troops to offset boredom, reduce mental stress, improve fitness, help with sleep, and increase energy. He feels it is a way to reduce the negative effects of adrenaline that is elevated in the stressful combat environment. In addition it will make the time of the tour go faster and keep the troops out of trouble. He notes that the military contracts for KP duties. He thinks it could save money and keep troops busy with these mundane tasks if it would assign them to the enlisted men instead of hiring others to do the work.

Medications and Biological Advances

Positron emission tomography (PET) scans have helped us understand the areas of the brain that are affected by combat stress and the neurological mechanisms that lead to the symptoms of PTSD. The diagnostic examinations have become more sophisticated and permit us to diagnose veterans suffering from PTSD with 95 percent accuracy. When we were in Vietnam, our combat stress patients would arrive sandwiched between two stretchers on the side of a helicopter. We used Thorazine and Mellaril for *dauerschlaft* techniques in which we sedated soldiers with combat stress reactions. We treated them with a shower, rest, good food, and supportive counseling with the expectancy they would return to their units, and we put them in contact with their comrades, who kidded them and welcomed them back. Typically two soldiers from the patient's unit would come to the clearing station to retrieve him. They'd comment how he was a gold brick and ask if we had round-eyed nurses. They'd take him back to their unit and let him know that he was still one of them. In the recent conflicts, the medicines have improved. The serotonin reuptake inhibitors (SSRIs) like Zoloft and Paxil are more effective for PTSD. Inderal, a beta-blocker used commonly in civilian practice for hypertension and, in lower doses, for intention tremor, has also been shown to be helpful with acute stress reactions. Soldiers treated in the combat zone with Inderal may be protected from problems later on. These drugs are more effective than those we employed in Vietnam and safer as well. Future medications will become more specific and effective in years to come. For example, an enzyme, Cdk5, which is modified in the hippocampus of the brain, may yield possibilities for the future treatment of PTSD. When this enzyme is blocked in rats, their memory of a traumatic experience is blocked as well. Should this translate into human experience it might be possible to block out the memories of traumatic events. By the way, the hippocampus is part of the limbic system or the primitive (lizard) brain. It is not, as one nonmedical person suggested, a large campus.

The military has recently developed a blood test that detects proteins released from damaged brain cells. This test can be used to support the diagnosis of mTBI and TBI.

The objective tests for PTSD and for TBI will go a long way toward developing more specific treatments, supporting legitimate disability claims, and reducing the stigma that still exists in the minds of many regarding these combat-related injuries.

The VA has recently authorized the use of expensive, long-acting, intramuscularly injected atypical antipsychotic medications in an effort to reduce the number of homeless veterans who are on the streets. They note that a large percentage of the homeless population is made up of individuals with chronic mental illnesses and that their symptoms are frequently reduced with antipsychotic medication. These patients are unwilling or unable to take oral medicines on a regular basis, but they can tolerate biweekly or monthly injections. Invega and Risperdal Consta are two IM long-acting atypical medicines that have been found to be particularly effective for this population.

An Application for Smartphones

Walter Reed and CTIS Inc. in Rockville are working together to develop an application for warriors with PTSD called mWarrior.

Support from Home

This is one area where we have been doing a good job. There are many organizations, websites, and programs to help veterans and their families. This not to say they couldn't use more assistance.

CSM Huber brought the State Farm Insurance Company Military Affinity Group (MAG) to my attention. CMS Huber helped start this program, which helps returning veterans find jobs in the company. It also sends letters, goodies, and items to military members that they can pass on to Iraqi and Afghan citizens and their children. For example, State Farm has all sorts of items it give to its agents for professional promotion (notepads, pens, umbrellas, towels, yo-yos, etc.). The company sells these items at cost to MAG, which sends cases of them to soldiers to pass out to locals. MAG publishes a newsletter with articles about soldiers and their families, encouraging employees to support them during deployment. Many other companies have similar programs for veterans. For example, J. C. Penney provides suits for veterans to wear when they are applying for civilian jobs after deployment. The Wounded Warrior program asks civilians to donate $19.95 a month to support injured veterans and their families. Admiral Mike Mullen, chairman of the Joint Chiefs of Staff, has been speaking publicly around the country, urging companies and communities to support our returning veterans and their families.

Compensation

One topic that is largely ignored in the literature is that of compensation and the effect that this has on the development and recovery from psychological-induced combat disability. A few years ago I was in the loo of a local pub in England, standing at a urinal when a Beefeater came in and stood at the next stall. "You a Yank?" he asked. I said I was. "You a vet?" he inquired. Again, I answered in the affirmative. "Your country doesn't do much for its vets," he commented. He then proceeded to tell me about all of the benefits English veterans receive from their government. He got me thinking, and I had to agree we don't do enough for our veterans. My father-in-law was in the Bataan Death March and was a prisoner of war for three and a half years in Japan and never received a penny from the government. Some would point out that he didn't request any help, but it would seem to me that he was certainly entitled to some compensation, and the fact that he was too proud to ask for it should not have prevented his receiving some aid.

Conservative commentator Rush Limbaugh pointed out some of the inequities in the way we compensate our military personnel. Families of individuals who were killed on 9/11 received $250,000 to $4.7 million, for an average of $1,185,000. A surviving family member of an American soldier killed in action receives a $6,000 death benefit, half of which is taxable, and $1,750 for burial costs. A surviving spouse receives $833/month until he or she remarries. Children receive $211/month until they reach eighteen. Members of Congress who have served only one term receive a pension of over $15,000/month. They do not pay into the Social Security system. Military who stay in for twenty years and get out as an E-7 may receive $1,000/month. Think about that: The soldiers who volunteer to be put in harm's way receive $1,000/month pension after twenty years of service. Those who vote to put them in harm's way receive $15,000/month after four years of service.

Dr. Hoge, in his book *Once a Warrior—Always a Warrior*, notes disability is a Catch-22 situation. Veterans have to be sick enough to qualify for compensation and yet well enough to get through the significant paperwork hurdles that application for benefits requires. My thinking is that anyone who served in a combat zone who develops psychological difficulties should be taken at his or her word and offered treatment. One problem with this is the problem of feigning or malingering. B. G. Burkett and Glenna Whitely wrote their now-classic book, *Stolen Valor*, to expose a number of famous cases of individuals who falsely claimed to have served in Vietnam. There have been a number of similar instances of politicians and others who have publicly lied about their combat service and who were subsequently exposed.

We had this experience in the First Infantry Division in Vietnam. We often attended a monthly psychiatric case conference at the Ninety-third Evacuation Hospital in Long Binh. We would don our flak jackets, helmets, and weapons and drive to Long Binh for what to us was an in-country rest and recuperation (R&R). We looked forward to visiting the Chinese restaurant and steam bath located on the post. One morning we walked into the conference a little late. One of the hospital psychiatrists had been interviewing an enlisted man from the First Infantry Division in front of an audience of psychiatrists, psychiatric social workers, psychologists, nurses, medics, and technicians. The patient, Private First Class Walker (pseudonym), had identified himself as 11 Bravo (infantryman). He'd been telling the audience and his interviewer that, after seeing his best buddy killed before his eyes, he'd started drinking to cope with the shock and grief he was experiencing. He told how his condition had deteriorated to the point where he'd been sent to the evacuation

VIII. Ideas for the Future

hospital. The audience was sympathetic and wanted to medically evacuate him out of country, feeling he had suffered enough. The interviewer saw us enter the room and said, "Here's Major Bey from the First Infantry. Let's have him interview the patient." I went up on stage and PFC Walker noted my First Infantry Division patch.

Bey: "What's your MOS?"
Walker: "11 Bravo, sir."
Bey: "Where were you assigned?"
Walker: "Headquarters Company, sir."
Bey: "What did you do there?"
Walker: "Deliver the mail, sir."

A murmur went through the audience at this point.

Bey: "How did you ever see anyone get killed while you were delivering mail at headquarters?"

Walker: "Well, no, sir, I didn't actually see anyone get killed—I just heard that he got killed."

By this time the audience realized that they had been duped and wanted to punish the soldier. Eventually they calmed down and sent him back to the division to continue delivering the mail. This interview convinced me of the need to have psychiatrists in combat divisions. REMFs in Long Binh believed the soldier's war stories. They were glad they weren't in the field but felt guilty about having a relatively safe assignment while others served in more dangerous and less comfortable settings. The soldier played on their guilt and controlled them in this way. By implicitly asserting that the audience members lived in comfortable surroundings and had no idea of what "hell" he had been through, he played on their sympathy to persuade them to send him home. It is similar to a panhandler confronting passersby with his handicap and playing on their guilt to get money. If an REMF assigned to delivering mail at the First Infantry Division headquarters could do this to mental health professionals serving in Vietnam, one can only imagine how someone claiming to be a Vietnam veteran could manipulate mental health professionals back in the United States. The ability to use guilt to manipulate others continues to this day in the legacy of imposters who claim to have been traumatized while serving in Vietnam. In *Stolen Valor*, Burkett and Whitley describe how men with long hair, fatigues, boots, and boonie hats portray themselves as the crazy, drugged-out, violent stereotype many people have of Vietnam veterans to garner sympathy, attention, and disability compensation. By researching government records, they show how many of these people either never served in Vietnam or served in a support capacity such as cooks or clerks. I once saw a guy walking through a shopping mall at home with a jacket that read, "When I die I will go to heaven because I spent a year in hell—Long Binh 1969–1970." To the REMFs who served in a combat division support command such as Di An, Long Binh was considered pretty close to heaven. My personal experience is that most people who tell war stories back in the United States are probably full of it. I have seen guys who started to tell war stories admit to serving as cooks or clerks and not having any direct combat experience once they learned that I had been in Vietnam. My father-in-law survived the Bataan Death March during World War II and was a Japanese prisoner of war for over three years. He did not talk about his experiences. Typically, Vietnam veterans rarely mention they served there. Some, if they know I was there, will talk about it a little. Over the years I've seen Vietnam "wannabes" who told war stories about the trauma they experienced although they never served in Vietnam. One such case was the second husband of one of my patients. Her first husband had been killed tragically in an accident. She later met a man in a bar who almost immediately told her that he was a Vietnam veteran. She brought him to an appointment and introduced him to my head nurse and me. The man told us how he had been wounded when his helicopter had been shot down, and that he crawled to the edge of the jungle and watched the Vietcong kill his crewmates. He had several other exciting adventures, which he described in detail. My head nurse, Eric Traub, RN, MSN, who served with the Eighty-Second Airborne Division in Vietnam, and I discussed the stories after he left. At first we were sympathetic, but as the descriptions of his exploits continued and escalated, we began to suspect that the guy was full of crap. A few months later, the fellow's wife noticed he didn't have any scars although he described being wounded by bullets and shrapnel. He said that they had healed. She asked his mother when he was in Vietnam. She responded that he was never in Vietnam. Needless to say, it strains credibility to have someone brag about his war experience to women in bars and to therapists but never tell his mother. When his wife confronted him with his mother's statement, he replied that he had been on a secret mission and no one knew he was there. During our sympathetic phase, we paid the man to serve as our office Santa Claus at our annual Christmas party. He arrived late, obviously intoxicated, but did a great job with the kids and played the part well—he was a good actor. The point being that good actors will have no problem telling their war stories to those in the rear and, especially, to those at home who have never served in combat. The men who served in the veteran's unit during the same period are best able to evaluate the individual's accounts of his combat experience.

Suggestibility, Placebo Effect, Secondary Gain, Malingering, and Fair Compensation

These are topics that are not usually discussed but are certainly present and affect the expression of symptoms and the chronicity of illness.

Suggestibility and Placebo Effect

The young military population is, in general, quite suggestible. This is probably a factor in the rapid instillation of new behaviors during basic and individual training. Some examples of this in the military:

At Ireland Army Hospital at Fort Knox, Kentucky, we had a busload of new recruits arrive at the emergency room, all hyperventilating. Apparently one trainee started panicking in the barracks, and the next thing every soldier in the barracks was overbreathing and passing out. We ran out of paper bags to have them breathe into.

A prisoner from the stockade showed up at the ER with stomach pain, and an x-ray revealed a double-edged razor blade in his stomach. He was admitted by surgery for observation, and soon there were eighteen more prisoners in the ER with razor blades in their stomachs. The surgeon called me and said we should admit them to psychiatry. I declined, indicating that should we do this, we would have the whole stockade admitted to the hospital. I suggested two plans: 1. We admit one prisoner to the top floor of the hospital and then spread the word at the stockade that he died. Or 2. We keep the prisoners at the stockade and observe them there. The surgeon opted for #2, and the new cases of razor swallowing ended. We later found that one prisoner had learned the technique of wrapping a razor blade in toilet paper and then swallowing it at another stockade. It was a means to escape from the stockade to the hospital for a brief respite. However, as the other prisoners soon witnessed, it was painful, and then the individual finally passed the razor blade.

On the positive side, suggestibility probably speeds training and indoctrination of new behavioral patterns needed to become a warrior. It can speed healing. Solomon's principles of military psychiatry from World War I included "expectancy" in which the caregivers provided a milieu for the individual with shell shock that conveyed an expectancy that the individual would quickly recover. On the negative side, talking about an illness can produce it. For example, in the 1970s suicide prevention programs were held in high schools to try to lower the incidence of teenage suicides. The program had the opposite effect, and the rates went up. The program was discontinued. The Columbine shootings led to a rash of copycat school shootings. No doubt the current publicity surrounding the increasing rates of suicide among the troops and the incidence of PTSD are also a factor in their growing numbers.

Secondary Gain

This is gain that comes as the result of having the illness. For example, when we admitted a patient air evacuated from Vietnam with hysterical symptoms, we would institute a specific treatment plan. The medics on the psychiatric unit would tell the individual that he would be given sodium amytal at the end of the week, which would help him recall and verbalize the psychological conflicts that caused his symptoms. The patient would be instantly cured and would then go on a pass home for thirty days. If, for some reason, the person was not cured, we would know that his problems were not due to unconscious psychological conflicts, and he would be retained in the hospital for further evaluation and testing. He would also be exposed to other cured patients who would attest to the wonders of our treatment efforts. At the end of the week, the patient would be brought to a darkened room where I would enter in my starched lab coat and give him the sodium amytal. We had a 100 percent cure rate, often as soon as the needle touched patients' skin. The same technique worked in Vietnam, but we, like Dr. Grinker in World War II, were never able to return them to combat duty. When we tried to send them back to the field, their symptoms returned.

In these cases individuals were in a combat area where they feared for their lives but were also afraid to run from their units or the dangerous situations they were in. Instead they became paralyzed, mute, lost their sight or their hearing, and had to be evacuated from danger to a medical facility. Once there, their symptoms persisted because to drop them would mean a return to combat and/or admission that they had escaped danger and were OK physically. In other words, they were in conflict between fearing for their lives and wanting to leave the combat area and not wanting to be cowardly or let down their comrades. The hysterical symptom solved the conflict by getting them out of danger but in an honorable way—due to physical limitations. To get rid of the symptom, the person's honor had to be protected, and we offered the secondary gain of a thirty-day leave to those patients evacuated to Fort Knox. The ones in Vietnam had the secondary gain of being reassigned to a rear area.

These factors come into play when veterans return home after deployment. To drop their symptoms, they may have to face their survival guilt of having made it home without being injured or killed. They may have to face demands they don't want to face. Compensation is involved where symptoms are rewarded with disability checks from the VA. I recall, as a medical student and later as a psychiatric resident, seeing VA patients experience a recurrence of their auditory hallucinations when they were reevaluated at the VA for the purpose of reviewing their disability ratings. If their symptoms abated, so would their monthly disability checks. In civilian practice, two-thirds of PTSD patients respond to treatment, but in the two largest VA studies there was no improvement. Most veterans getting PTSD treatment at VA facilities report worsening symptoms until they are rated 100 percent disabled, and then their use of the VA mental health services drop by 82 percent. The same phenomenon occurs with the diagnosis of TBI. Ninety-nine percent of cases of TBI are mild (mTBI) or a concussion, which should recover quickly with no treatment. Unfortunately, these are lumped in with TBI, which refers to traumatic, usually permanent, brain damage. Because of our current system of compensation, the headaches, memory problems, and emotional labiality that becomes associated with both diagnoses persists because failure to do so would result in the loss of approximately $2,800/month by the veteran. Recovery also means an end to the associated benefits of free medication and medical care. There are also benefits for the surviving spouse of the disabled veteran. This system tends to lead to chronic disability.

I don't believe these situations represent conscious malingering in most cases but, rather, an unconscious response on the patients' part. My professor Karl Menninger had a unique view of malingering in his book *The Vital Balance:*

"There is another type of personality deformity which is so ancient and classical, so commonly assumed to be prevalent, and yet so rare, that we must list it out of sheer curiosity. It is the compulsive deception represented by the feigning of disease. Curiously enough, the individual who does this, the malingerer, does not himself believe that he is ill, but tries to persuade others that he is, and they discover, they think, that he is not ill, but the sum of all this, in the opinion of myself and my perverse-minded colleagues, is precisely that he is ill, in spite of what others think. No healthy-minded person would go to such extremes and take such devious and painful routes for minor gains that the invalid status brings to the malingerer."

Dr. Karl demonstrated this while on rounds with us on the psychiatric service of the Winter VA Hospital in Topeka, Kansas. The hospital had a swimming pool, a gym, a canteen, a theater, and many other pleasant features for the patients. The patients were collecting 100 percent disability while residing in the hospital. One of the residents commented, "Well, who wouldn't like to be a patient here and have all these benefits while collecting a nice check?" Dr. Karl said that he had some influence with the hospital and he would see to it that the resident was admitted to the service the next morning.

The resident stammered and started backpedaling. "I didn't mean that I personally wanted to be in the hospital. I have a wife and family." "No," replied Dr. Karl, "you said anyone would like to be in the hospital, so pack your bag and be here for admission tomorrow morning." The resident continued to protest, and Dr. Karl finally let him off of the hook and said, "You see, no one who is really not ill would want to stay in the hospital."

One problem for the VA is the aging veteran population. Median ages by period of service are: Gulf War, thirty-seven years old; Vietnam War, sixty (representing 7.9 million and the largest portion of the veteran population); Korean War, seventy-six; and World War II, eighty-four. The percentage of the veteran population over sixty-five is 39.1 percent. The demand for medical services increases with age—7.2 million veterans are enrolled in the VA system, 5.5 million receive health care, and 3.4 million receive benefits.

The VA has been criticized for having a backlog of six hundred thousand disability payments and delays up to 177 days for initial claims. A memo was discovered that instructed VA professionals to use diagnoses such as "adjustment reaction" rather than PTSD, presumably to reduce the number of veterans eligible for compensation. Following their deployment to OEF and OIF, 1,019 marines charged with misconduct were discharged under less than honorable conditions. This meant that they would receive no military benefits (no disability, no VA treatment, no GI Bill, etc.). A follow-up study showed that 326 of these men had significant mental health problems, and the question arose whether they might have been discharged in this manner to avoid giving them compensation later on. Another study noted that the military was administratively discharging ten soldiers/day under less than honorable conditions for preexisting personality problems. The VA has hired more than 3,800 mental health workers since 2005 and has a total mental health workforce of nearly seventeen thousand employees. In 2007 there was one mental

VIII. Ideas for the Future

health practitioner for every 734 soldiers. The mental health services of the military are overwhelmed with the soldiers who do ask for help. There is a concern that many professionals suffer from "compassion fatigue." There is also concern that due to the great need for help and the shortage of professionals available, the military may not be screening the quality of its professional mental health caregivers adequately because of desperation to try to meet the demand. Critics point to Major Nidal Hasan and how, seemingly, his ideology and poor performance were ignored by the military prior to his gunning down thirteen soldiers at Fort Hood.

Use the Treatment Modalities That Are Most Effective, Least Expensive, and Most Accessible

The current literature suggests that self-managed cognitive behavioral therapy (SM-CBT) is effective for PTSD when presented as an eight-week course online. This offers a viable treatment modality that is inexpensive and easily accessible in the privacy of the veteran's home. This bypasses the concerns about confidentiality, cost, career, and security clearance problems. These resistances are currently problems that get in the way of many veterans receiving help. One study suggested that 70 percent of military respondents thought they would be labeled as being "crazy" if they sought mental health assistance, and the majority felt fellow workers would judge them negatively if they knew they were receiving mental health assistance.

Common Sense Versus Red Tape

I can recall older doctors describing medical practice prior to Medicaid. The newest doctors in town would accept indigent patients. They wanted to see patients and had plenty of time available. They would charge their usual fees but have an understanding with the patients that they would pay what they could on the bill and the doctor would carry the balance and not press them for payment. This made the doctor feel good for being able to help others, and the patient was grateful to the physician. Then Medicaid came into existence. The patient was given a green card and told it would take care of all medical bills. Layers of government workers used up money for the program, so little remained when it came to paying the doctors. The physician received a small amount of compensation as before, but in many cases he was now confronted with a demanding, ungrateful patient. The taxpayers were burdened by another wasteful government program.

Another similar situation comes to mind. A fellow in a small town near here became ill and unable to work. One of the township supervisors went to his house and said that the town was aware of his illness and would pay his house payment and provide him with money for groceries and utilities for three months until he got back on his feet. He added that the township expected he would repay this money when he regained his health. The man was grateful and did repay the money after he recovered. I give this as an example of how much better it is to have a personal relationship with a person in need rather than a big government program sending an impersonal check. Also, it demonstrates that expectation of recovery and repayment of money provided during infirmity is possible rather than encouraging disability and dependency on the system as we seem to have a tendency do.

Thinking Outside the Box

From the statistics cited earlier in the book, it appears that current approaches to mental health in the military and for veterans are not working. Increasing numbers of mental health problems, suicides, chemical dependency, and traumatic brain injuries are being reported. A large proportion of soldiers with problems fail to seek professional help. The available services are overwhelmed by the demands of those who do ask for assistance. There are concerns about the quality of the professionals recruited by the government to supply the need. Veterans tell me of delays in receiving help from

VIII. Ideas for the Future

the VA and what seems to be an adversarial relationship in which they have to beg for more compensation for their problems while the VA tries to give them as little as possible. Many complain that the professionals they see have not had combat or even military experience and do not seem to understand their complaints.

The current system of compensation frequently leads to permanent invalidism. In addition to the problems receiving medical attention and compensation, a large number of veterans are unemployed and many are homeless. Programs like BATTLEMIND and resiliency training may be of some help to individual soldiers, but they are baby steps when it comes to changing today's escalating trend of mental problems among returning veterans. The same goes for virtual reality, balance training, and other technologically based interventions for PTSD and TBI.

It appears we need to step back from the current approaches to these problems and look at them in a different way. What do we really mean by "thinking outside the box"? Two examples from medical school come to mind. One question on the neuroanatomy final in medical school was: "Arrange the following neurological structures in any meaningful order." A list of neuroanatomical structures was then given. We listed them in order of their anatomical arrangement in the body or physiologically according to function. One student in our class of two hundred wrote "alphabetical" and listed them in according to their starting letters. He was given full credit for his answer, and the rest of us wondered why we had been so dumb to overlook this simple approach. A second humorous example also occurred during my medical school days. Dr. Max Samter was a professor of endocrinology. He presented a young male patient with gynecomastia (enlarged breasts). The breasts were lactating (secreting milk). Next he introduced us to a young man with juvenile diabetes. He then asked us to correlate the two cases. We talked about the pituitary as the master gland and the possible connections between the symptoms exhibited by the two patients. "No, no," said Dr. Samter. "You don't get it. First I show you a man who makes milk, then I show you one who makes sugar. If we find one who makes coffee, we're in business!"

It seems we need to attempt step out of our old thought patterns when it comes to mental health problems in the military and our veterans.

A Radical Proposal—Reward Health and Recovery

I think the English Beefeater I met in the London pub's loo was right when he said that Yanks don't do enough for their veterans. I feel that all veterans who served in combat should be recognized and compensated for their service in some way. Currently those who are disabled and their spouses receive money and medical benefits (medicines paid for, and their widows receive compensation). Combat veterans who adjust to civilian life and fail to claim disability do not receive any benefits. I believe disabled veterans should receive disability compensation, but the current system rewards and encourages chronic disability and invalidism. In the big picture, if you reward people who are not productive with compensation and benefits and penalize those who work with taxes, you will eventually destroy individual incentive to work hard and be productive.

I witnessed this years ago in Australia, where citizens were taxed at 90 percent for any income over $10,000. People would earn up to $10,000 and then quit working. A plumber in Sydney told me he could have twenty-five plumbers working for him and keep them all busy, "But what's the point? The government takes it all." He worked alone and quit when he got close to $10,000. Physicians were no different. They worked on salary at government hospitals with long lunch hours and what we would call a very easy schedule. They said they could have all the private patients they wanted, but again, they would be essentially working for nothing and turning everything over to the government. One doctor who raised purebred cattle said the year he sold his cattle he didn't work as a psychiatrist because he would have given 90 percent of what he earned to the government.

My proposal would be to continue to compensate and provide benefits for combat veterans who are disabled. But, in addition, those who successfully made the adjustment from the war zone to civilian life would be rewarded as well. I would suggest that all veterans who served in a combat zone receive combat pension and medical benefits that would be equal or more than they could receive if they were 100 percent disabled. Veterans receiving disability could have the choice whether they would prefer receiving disability compensation or combat veteran's compensation. This would allow many to recover from their disabilities without loss of income and reduce the stigma for seeking help. (Many disabled veterans do not make the effort to receive disability because they feel as though they are begging for a handout.) In addition, as mentioned earlier, all returning veterans would be required to see a counselor for a prescribed number of sessions. This program would be akin to police officers being required to see a therapist after being involved in a shooting on the job. This would overcome the resistance many veterans have to seeking help for themselves as well as the stigma connected with mental health treatment.

Combat veterans who demonstrated a successful adjustment after combat service could be trained and hired as mentors and peer counselors to provide the required therapy services to returning veterans. These trained peer counselors could also see returning veterans still struggling with the postdeployment adaptation. This would provide full or part-time employment and additional income for many veterans. Other combat veterans could be hired to conduct peer reviews of claims submitted by veterans who served in their combat units during the same period overseas.

They would be empathetic and would lean toward supporting the veteran's need for compensation, but they would also be able to weed out individuals who were feigning combat experience. Take as an example the mailman I saw in Vietnam who said he saw his buddy blown up. A veteran who served in the same unit at about the same time would remember the incident and may have witnessed it himself. He would be in the best position to support the returning warrior's claim or to recognize that he was malingering. If the case was appealed, another veteran from the unit could be asked for an opinion.

In addition, couples whose marriages and families weathered the stress of deployment could be hired and compensated to mentor new couples and help them deal with the stresses of being married in the military. Spouses who coped with their warrior's deployment(s) could be hired as mentors and serve as role models for spouses new to the military.

Finally, experienced NCOs, commanding officers, and medical officers who are retired or discharged from the military could be utilized to consult with units regarding problems that are producing stress in the units. They could function as civilian consultants and could use modern technology like videoconferencing to give on-the-spot advice to commanders in the field.

The military is struggling to recruit and retain mental health professionals to meet the increasing demands for mental health services at home and also among combat troops overseas. Veterans are having difficulties finding employment. Perhaps by training healthy veterans, healthy spouses, and experienced veterans these needs could be met, and the healthy individuals who coped with the stresses of deployment would be rewarded as well. One Special Forces veteran pointed out that counseling might bring up the veteran's own problems from combat. I agree, but, as with Alcoholics

VIII. Ideas for the Future

Anonymous or other self-help groups, this may be therapeutic for the healthy veteran as well.

Training and utilizing combat veterans and their spouses, as well as retirees, would provide additional income and employment for many veterans and their families. As of publication, the US civilian unemployment rate is over 9 percent while the unemployment rate of veterans is 12 percent. Veterans and their families who coped with deployment and a normal return to civilian life would be rewarded. Health, recovery, and positive family outcomes would be recognized and compensated. Utilizing retired and discharged military personnel to counsel combat commanders would provide an untapped reservoir of wisdom and experience that could be utilized to help lower the stress of troops in battle. The military and the VA are having difficulty recruiting and retaining professionals to meet the mental health needs of soldiers, returning veterans, and their families. They are also having problems finding mental health consultants to meet the needs of troops in the field. There have been questions about the quality of some of the professionals they've had to accept. Utilizing individuals who have made the adjustments successfully and who have been leaders in combat to mentor and consult would meet the need for mental health caregivers and also reduce some of the stresses experienced by combat units in the field. This approach may also lead to changes in our current veterans disability system. As we've seen, under the current programs, disability is compensated and recovery leads to a loss of income for the veteran and his or her family. In other words, disability is rewarded and recovery is penalized. By rewarding health, veterans would no longer feel penalized by recovery from their disabilities. The government would save the money it was paying for chronic invalidism in many cases. Utilizing veterans and their spouses as mentors and counselors would represent a cost savings and would solve the government's inability to recruit and retain sufficient numbers of professional mental health workers. This approach would also help reduce the high rate of unemployment among veterans.

Our future security depends on our warriors and the support of their families. We need to encourage and support them. We should advocate for them by contacting our elected representatives. Members of the military and their loved ones need and deserve additional compensation for their sacrifices on our behalf.

IX Postscript

In conclusion, our warriors are one of our nation's greatest assets. Eighty-five percent of troops are considered support troops and 15 percent are outside of the wire kicking in doors, disarming IEDs, shooting enemy troops, and being shot at themselves. This elite minority of the troops is the tip of the sword, highly trained, and highly motivated. As of 2007, one-third of troops have served two tours in a combat area, seventy thousand three times, and twenty thousand have been deployed at least five times. Support troops were not safe from danger. They were exposed to rockets, mortars, IEDs, VBIEDs, and suicide bombers. Support troops are exposed to adverse climatic conditions, separation from their families, and the unique stresses of a hardship assignment. Despite the dangers and stresses our troops and their families endure, most military families adjust without professional help. This book was written to provide advice to help ease their adaptation and to assist those with more severe problems receive the best possible aid that is currently available.

In general, it behooves our warriors and their families to maintain a positive attitude. You are the best-trained, most intelligent, and best fighting men and women ever. Your country is proud of you and supports you. Most of you continue to cope with your stressful lives without help. Ignore the negative picture presented by the media. As I was leaving a dermatologist's office, he said,

"Stay out of the sun." "Why," I asked, "do I have a problem that requires me to avoid the sun?" "No," he answered, "I say that to all of my patients—don't you have something in psychiatry that you say to all of your patients?" I thought for a moment and then answered, "Well, how about don't watch the news?" Too much exposure to news broadcasts these days can, in my opinion, lead to a negative outlook and depression. In contrast to the media, I believe it would help all of us to dwell on the positive events in our lives and to be thankful for our many blessings. Pay attention to the miracles that happen to us. My advice to our military heroes is to be proud of your service and the sacrifices you have made for the rest of us. We are grateful and you are in our thoughts and prayers.

As with any precious commodity, we need to protect, support, and nurture our warriors for the future survival of our country. As we watched the rescue of the thirty-three miners in Chili recently, I was struck by the thought that these men survived the isolation, danger, adverse conditions, and boredom of sixty-nine days underground. Our troops survive 365 days or more of adverse conditions, danger, and boredom in the cultural isolation of a combat assignment. Shouldn't we celebrate and support their safe return with as much energy and joy as the world showed the miners? The miners were provided six months of psychological treatment after their sixty-nine-day ordeal. Shouldn't our veterans receive that much and more? These are our heroes, and the rest of us who have benefited from their courage and self-sacrifice should do all we can to honor and support them. Their families have sacrificed, usually unnoticed, and deserve our gratitude and support as well.

I've interviewed many men and a few women who endured multiple dangerous combat experiences. When I point out their obvious heroism, they all say the same thing: "The real heroes are underground."

IX Postscript

Just because they remain humble and deny their heroism doesn't mean that we should. I think we should make an effort to recognize and honor our returning veterans' bravery and advocate for benefits for them as a token of our nation's gratitude for their service. Let your elected representatives know you support financial support for soldiers and their families.

Pray for our warriors and their loved ones. Thank them for their service when you have an opportunity to do so. We are obligated to do all we can for our nation's heroes.

Most veterans live quiet lives and pass away mourned only by their friends and families.

He was getting old and paunchy
and his hair was falling fast,
and he sat around the Legion,
telling stories of the past.

Of a war that he once fought in
and the deeds that he had done,
in his exploits with his buddies;
they were heroes, every one.

And 'tho sometimes to his neighbors
his tales became a joke,
all his buddies listened quietly
for they knew where of he spoke.

But we'll hear his tales no longer,
for Ol' Jim has passed away,
and the world's a little poorer
for a Soldier died today.

Supporting You and Your Combat Veteran During and After Deployment

He won't be mourned by many,
just his children and his wife.
for he lived an ordinary,
very quiet sort of life.

He held a job and raised a family,
going quietly on his way;
and the world won't note his passing,
'tho a Soldier died today.

When politicians leave this earth,
their bodies lie in state,
while thousands note their passing,
and proclaim that they were great.

Papers tell of their life stories
from the time that they were young,
but the passing of a Soldier
goes unnoticed, and unsung.

Is the greatest contribution
to the welfare of our land,
some jerk who breaks his promise
and cons his fellow man?

Or the ordinary fellow
who in times of war and strife,
goes off to serve his country
and offers up his life?

The politician's stipend
and the style in which he lives,
are often disproportionate,
to the service that he gives.

IX Postscript

While the ordinary Soldier,
who offered up his all,
is paid off with a medal
and perhaps a pension, small.

It is not the politicians
with their compromise and ploys,
who won for us the freedom
that our country now enjoys.

Should you find yourself in danger,
with your enemies at hand,
would you really want some cop-out,
with his ever-waffling stand?

Or would you want a Soldier—
his home, his country, his kin,
just a common Soldier,
who would fight until the end.

He was just a common Soldier,
and his ranks are growing thin,
but his presence should remind us
we may need his like again.

For when countries are in conflict,
we find the Soldier's part,
is to clean up all the troubles
that the politicians start.

If we cannot do him honor
while he's here to hear the praise,
then at least let's give him homage
at the ending of his days.

Perhaps just a simple headline
in the paper that might say:

"OUR COUNTRY IS IN MOURNING,
A SOLDIER DIED TODAY."

— Anonymous

A Soldier

I was that which others did not wish to be.

I went where others feared to go and did what others failed to do.

I asked nothing from those who gave nothing and reluctantly accepted the thought of eternal loneliness…should I fail.

I have seen the face of terror: felt the stinging cold of fear and enjoyed the sweet taste of moments of love.

I have cried, pained, and hoped…but most of all I have lived times others would say were best forgotten.

At least someday I will be able to say that I was proud of what I was…a soldier.

Anonymous

X References

Personal Accounts

Of Deployment in OIF:

Hartley, Jason Christopher. *Just Another Soldier: A Year on the Ground in Iraq.* New York, London, Toronto, Sydney: Harper, 2003, 238.

One young soldier's account of his tour in Iraq. A diary of the experience of service in Iraq.

Crawford, John. *The Last True Story I'll Ever Tell: An Accidental Soldier's Account of the War in Iraq.* New York: Riverhead Books, 2005, 220.

An on-the-ground story of a member of the National Guard who was activated one semester short of graduating from college and newly married. He describes his experiences serving in the hostile city of Baghdad. Like the book above, it will give families a day-to-day idea of what their loved one experienced during his deployment.

Buzzell, Colby. *My War: Killing Time in Iraq.* New York: Berkley Caliber, 2005, 358.

A personal account of a machine gunner's tour in Iraq.

Combat in Afghanistan (OEF):

Junger, Sebastian. *War*. New York: Hachette Book Group, 2010.

A war correspondent describes the experience of combat in Afghanistan. An excellent book to understand what soldiers at the tip of the sword in Afghanistan experienced during their deployment there.

Of Combat in World War II and Other Wars:

Sajer, Guy. *The Forgotten Soldier: A Classic German WWII Autobiography*. Washington, DC: Potomac Books Inc., 1971, 464.

A realistic description of the horrors of war on the Eastern front from the perspective of a foot soldier in an elite German infantry unit. The adverse climatic conditions, continuous battle, lack of air superiority, lack of equipment—these are stories of war as we've never experienced it.

Brown, Jesse, and Daniel Paisner. *The Price of Their Blood Profiles in Spirit*. Chicago and Los Angeles: Bonus Books, 2003, 221.

Heroes in battle who courageously overcame their disabilities to continue to contribute to others in life.

Sledge, E. B. *With the Old Breed*, 2010 Presidio Press Paperwork Edition, a division of Random House, copy 1981, 326.

Description of a Marine infantryman's experiences in the Pacific during World War II.

Leckie, Robert. *Helmet for My Pillow*. New York: Bantam Books, a division of Random House, copy 1957, 305.

A Marine in the Pacific during World War II gives an account of his experiences from training in Parris Island, South Carolina, to his experiences in war in the Pacific.

Marlantes, Karl. *Matterhorn.* New York: Atlantic Monthly Press, copy 2010.

A novel about a Marine unit in Vietnam. Well researched and a believable portrayal of combat in Vietnam.

Training Men to Kill and the Consequences of Taking a Life:

Grossman, Lt. Colonel Dave. *On Killing: The Psychological Cost of Learning to Kill in War and Society.* New York, Boston: Back Bay Books, Little Brown and Company, 1995, 366.

This is a Pulitzer Prize-nominated book. A scientific analysis of killing and the effect of killing one's own species on the soldier or police officer doing the killing. Colonel Grossman notes that this topic has largely been avoided by the military and the mental health workers trying to help veterans in the past. If we are going to condition soldiers and policemen to be capable of taking lives, we must also speak openly with them about the necessity and morality of their acts to help them avoid the guilt and suffering that follows. We need to help them see the lives they are saving as well as ending and the good their actions have caused. He discusses the associated guilt of those who didn't actually pull the trigger but supported those who did. In addition, he notes that we do in combat what we do in training and that we are training our youth through video games to become killers.

Grossman, Lt. Colonel Dave, with Loren W. Christensen. *On Combat: The Psychology and Physiology of Deadly Combat in War and in Peace.* Warrior Science Publications, printed in China, 2004, 403.

An analysis of combat. The physiologic changes that occur and how these influence perception in a life-and-death situation. How to remain clearheaded while faced with stress. Training to improve combat skills including the importance of continuing to fight after being shot. Lieutenant Colonel Grossman says there are warriors and there are sheep who follow orders. He observes that some men are resistant to kill but go ahead and do so on the basis that it is the right thing to do and it is necessary to protect our country and their comrades in arms. Others have no hesitation or second thoughts about killing. Neither group is wrong. There are also a few sociopaths who enjoy killing.

Klinger, David. *Into the Kill Zone: A Cop's Eye View of Deadly Force.* San Francisco: Jossey-Bass, A Wiley Imprint, 2004, 288.

A vivid description of combat situations and the perceptual changes that a policeman experiences under the stress of life-and-death situations.

Stone, Vali. *Cops Don't Cry: A Book of Help and Hope for Police Families.* Ontario, Canada: Creative Bound Inc., 1999, 234.

A description of the stresses innate in police work. Policemen's tendency to suppress and control their emotions and the problems that this causes in their marriages. Many parallels to the stresses experienced by combat soldiers can be seen.

Howe, MSG Paul R. Howe, US Army Ret. *Leadership and Training for the Fight: A Few Thoughts on Leadership and Training from a Former Special Operations Soldier.* Bloomington, Indiana: Author House, 2005, 197.

Practical advice on training leaders for soldiers, policemen, and business executives by an experienced special operations combat leader.

Holton, Chuck. *Bulletproof: The Making of an Invincible Mind.* Sisters, Oregon: Multnomah Publishers, 2005, 203.

A tough ranger teaches how a relationship with God can provide confidence in the face of adversity. Fear God and nothing else.

Siddle, Bruce K. *Sharpening the Warrior's Edge: The Psychology & Science of Training.* Belleville, Illinois: PPCT Management Systems, 1995, 148.

A discussion of combat training, including the physiologic and perceptual changes that occur in the stress of life-and-death situations.

Dyer, Gwynne. *War: The Lethal Custom.* New York: Carroll and Graf Publishers, 2005, 484.

A history of war and good description of how men are turned into killers by military training. Speculation as to whether mass communication and shared values might help us move beyond the need for war.

A DVD for Children

"Talk, Listen, Connect"

A DVD by Sesame Workshop and Wal-Mart to help children cope with their feelings during deployment.

A DVD Tracing the History of PTSD and War

Wartorn is a recent HBO documentary that traces the existence of stress disorders among soldiers starting with the ancient Greeks to present-day combat veterans.

Women in the Military

Williams, Kayla, with Michael E. Staub. *Love My Rifle More Than You: Young and Female in the U.S. Army.* New York, London: W. W. Norton & Co., 2005, 292.

A former female sergeant with the 101st Airborne Division describes the stresses of being one of a few females deployed with a majority of males in a combat zone.

Leyva, Meredith. *Married to the Military: A Survival Guide for Military Wives, Girlfriends, and Women in Uniform.* New York, London, Toronto, Sydney, Singapore: A Fireside Book, Simon and Schuster, 2003, 200.

Gutmann, Stephanie. *The Kinder, Gentler Military: How Political Correctness Affects Our Ability to Win Wars.* San Francisco: Encounter Books, 2000, 300.

How political correctness is undermining the aggression, competition, and respect for authority that has been part of a warrior culture.

Herbert, Melissa S. *Camouflage Isn't Only for Combat: Gender, Sexuality, and Women in the Military.* New York, London: New York University Press, 1995, 204.

Some of the problems facing women in the military. If they are feminine and friendly to the men, they are loose. If they hang out with the women, they are dykes.

Holmstedt, Kirsten. *Band of Sisters: American Women at War in Iraq.* Mechanicsburg, Pennsylvania: Stackpole Books, 2007, 327.

X References

Wise, James E. Jr., and Scott Baron. *Women at War Iraq: Afghanistan and Other Conflicts.* Annapolis, Maryland: Naval Institute Press, 2006, 234.

Description of courageous women serving in Afghanistan, Iraq, and other wars.

Skiba, Katherine M. *Sister in the Band of Brothers: Embedded with the 101st Airborne in Iraq.* University Press of Kansas, 1998, 257.

What it was like to be an embedded reporter in Iraq. Life in the base camps of Iraq.

Loss and Ambiguous Loss

Kubler-Ross, Elisabeth, MD. *On Death and Dying: What the Dying Have to Teach Doctors, Nurses, Clergy, and Their Own Families.* New York, London, Toronto, Sydney: Scribner, 1969, 285.

The application of Freud's *Mourning and Melancholia* to the stages of death. Very similar to the stages of loss described by Dr. Cholden below.

Cholden, Louis S. Cholden, MD., *A Psychiatrist Works with Blindness.* New York: American Foundation for the Blind, 1958, 119.

Dr. Cholden discusses the loss of sight on the basis of Freud's *Mourning and Melancholia.* It is very similar to the stages described by Dr. Kubler-Ross in her description of death.

Boss, Pauline. *Ambiguous Loss: Learning to Live with Unresolved Grief.* Cambridge, Massachusetts, London, England: Harvard University Press, 1999, 155.

Dr. Boss introduces the concept of ambiguous loss to describe situations where the person is emotionally unavailable and yet still alive. For example, a deployed soldier, a POW, an MIA, an addicted parent, a relative with Alzheimer's, a family permanently left in another country.

Boss, Pauline. *Loss, Trauma, and Resilience: Therapeutic Work with Ambiguous Loss.* New York, London: W. W. Norton & Company, 2006, 251.

Further discussion of ambiguous loss and its application in therapy.

Books on PTSD

Shay, Jonathan, MD, PhD. *Odysseus in America: Combat Trauma and the Trials of Homecoming.* New York, London, Toronto, Sydney, Singapore: Scribner, 2002, 329.

Utilizing Greek mythology to understand the warrior and applying the ancient wisdom to the treatment of veterans with PTSD.

Shay, Jonathan, MD, PhD. *Achilles in Vietnam: Combat Trauma and the Undoing of Character.* New York, London, Toronto, Sydney, Singapore: A Touchstone Book, Simon & Schuster, 1994, 246.

More experiences treating Vietnam veterans suffering from PTSD with parallels to ancient mythology.

Lanham, Stephanie Laite. *Veterans and Families' Guide to Recovering from PTSD.* Annandale, Virginia: Purple Heart Service Foundation, 2007, 118.

A small book filled with practical information for veterans and their families based on the author's extensive experience working with them.

X References

Hoge, Charles W. MD, Colonel US Army (Ret.). *Once a Warrior—Always a Warrior: Navigating the Transition from Combat to Home—Including Combat Stress, PTSD, and mTBI.* Guilford, Connecticut: GPP Life, an imprint of Globe Pequot Press, 2010, 303.

One of the best discussions of the effects of deployment and the adjustments by families and warriors during the postdeployment phase by an experienced military psychiatrist. The BATTLEMIND and resiliency programs instituted by the military are described.

Tick, Edward, PhD. *War and the Soul: Healing Our Nation's Veterans from Post-traumatic Stress Disorder.* Wheaton, Illinois, Chennai (Madras), India: Quest Books Theosophical Publishing House, 2005, 329.

Dr. Tick utilizes his extensive experience working with veterans with PTSD in a VA setting to describe his theory of healing the combat veteran's soul. His approach should be taken seriously in light of what we know about the effects of killing a member of one's own species on the combat soldier.

Matsakis, Aphrodite, PhD. *Vietnam Wives: Women and Children Surviving Life with Veterans Suffering Post Traumatic Stress Disorder.* Woodbine House, 1988, 423.

A psychologist with extensive experience working with veterans with PTSD.

Matsakis, Aphrodite, PhD. *Back from the Front: Combat Trauma, Love, and the Family.* Baltimore, Maryland: Sidran Institute Press, 2007, 478.

More clinical wisdom from a psychologist's experience working with veterans suffering from PTSD. Helping veterans and families adjust to one another after deployment.

Books for Veterans and Their Dependents on Deployment:

Edited by: Freeman, Sharon Morgillo, Bret A. Moore, and Arthur Freeman. *Living and Surviving in Harm's Way: A Psychological Treatment Handbook for Pre- and Post-Deployment of Military Personnel.* New York, London: Routledge Taylor & Francis Group, 2009, 513.

Excellent textbook for the professional who is working with military soldiers and their families.

Moore, Bret A., and Carrie H. Kennedy. *Wheels Down: Adjusting to Life After Deployment.* Washington D.C.: American Psychological Association, 2011, 184.

Advice for veterans and their families by two experienced military psychologists. Describes the common adjustment difficulties and the current suggested treatment.

Dumas, Alexander G., MD, and Grace Keen. *A Psychiatric Primer for the Veteran's Family and Friends.* Minneapolis: The University of Minnesota Press, 1945, 214.

Written in the 1940s to help returning World War II veterans in their families. It is interesting to know they faced the same adjustments back then.

Slone, Laurie B., PhD, and Matthew J. Friedman, MD, PhD. *After the War Zone: A Practical Guide for Returning Troops and Their Families.* Philadelphia: Da Capo Lifelong, A Member of the Perseus Books Group, 2008, 279.

An excellent in-depth look at the adjustments associated with military service, deployment, and readjustment to civilian life.

Sherman, Nancy. *The Untold War: Inside the Hearts, Minds, and Souls of Our Soldiers*. New York, London: W. W. Norton & Co., 2010, 338.

A deeper exploration of the moral aspects of military service and combat by a trained philosopher.

Cantrell, Bridget C., PhD, and Chuck Dean. *Down Range to Iraq and Back*. Seattle, Washington: Word Smith Publishing, 2005, 164.

Experiences in combat and the adjustment to civilian life postdeployment.

Cantrell, Bridget C., PhD, and Chuck Dean. *Once a Warrior: Wired for Life*. Seattle, Washington: Word Smith Publishing, 2007, 126.

Practical suggestions to help veterans make the adjustment back into civilian life.

Gaines, Tynisa. *Military Wives 101*. Bloomington, Indiana: 1st Books Library, 2002, 198.

A novel that describes the life of a military wife.

Martin, Hilary. *Solo-Ops: A Survival Guide for Military Wives*. Broomfield, Colorado: Xlibris Corporation, 2003, 240.

The author stresses the need for a sense of humor for a military spouse and demonstrates it in her writing. She prepares wives for the realities of military life and notes that the military is only giving lip service to its interest in wives and family because the organization found that, in order to retain servicemen, the wives had to be somewhat content with their lot.

Pavlicin, Karen M. *Surviving Deployment: A Guide for Military Families.* Saint Paul, Minnesota: Elva Resa Publishing, 2003, 288.

One of the best references for the waiting wife. Contains many practical lists and outlines for budgets that can be utilized. Also provides resources for support.

Pavlicin, Karen M. *Life After Deployment: Military Families Share Reunion Stories and Advice.* Saint Paul, Minnesota: Elva Resa Publishing, 2007, 180.

Stories by waiting wives that focus on the return and adjustment to being together again.

Hall, Lynn K. *Counseling Military Families: What Mental Health Professionals Need to Know.* New York, London: Routledge Taylor and Francis Group, 2008, 303.

An excellent book for professional counselors to help them understand the military culture and how to work with warriors and their families.

Cline, Lydia Sloan. *Today's Military Wife: Meeting the Challenges of Service Life.* Mechanicsburg, Pennsylvania: Stackpole Books, 2003, 3007.

Practical advice for the new military wife by an experienced military spouse. Information about resources and education about the military, including identifying rank, abbreviations, and proper etiquette.

Eckhart, Jacey. *The Homefront Club: The Hardheaded Woman's Guide to Raising a Military Family.* Annapolis, Maryland: Naval Institute Press, 2005, 224.

X References

Vandevoorde, Shellie. *Separated by Duty, United in Love: A Guide to Long-Distant Relationships for Military Couples.* Citadel Press, Kensington Publishing Group, 2003, 175.

Separations are stressful and can make or break your marriage. Help each other vent negative feelings. Support children and get into a routine. Don't feel sorry for yourself. Surround yourself with people who have good relationships with their spouses.

Henderson, Kristin. *While They're at War: The True Story of American Families on the Homefront.* Boston, New York: A Mariner Book, Houghton Mifflin Company, 2006, 317.

Discusses the experience of being a waiting wife and gives helpful, practical tips for wives to help them prepare and adjust to deployment and later to homecoming. She describes the stresses associated with life in the military and defines the stages of adjustment to deployment.

Biank, Tanya. *Under the Sabers: The Unwritten Code of Army Wives.* New York: St. Martin's Press, 2006, 260.

An army brat and journalist, the author goes into depth describing the lives of four army wives and their extraordinary stresses and sacrifices.

Kay, Ellie. *Heroes at Home: Help and Hope for America's Military Families.* Bloomington, Minnesota: Bethany House, 2002, 206.

Experiences of the spouse of an air force pilot who has been through numerous moves, raised five children, and endured deployments. Contains practical information regarding adjusting to the military culture, including terms and customs. Also many practical tips on keeping a budget.

Canfield, Jack, Mark Victor Hansen, Charles Preston, and Cindy Pedersen. *Chicken Soup for the Military Wife's Soul 10:1 Stories to Touch the Heart and Rekindle the Spirit.* Deerfield Beach, Florida: Health Communications Inc., 2003, 330.

Contains 101 short stories by military wives that describe their positive attitudes in the face of adversity and stress.

Vandesteeg, Carol. *When Duty Calls: A Handbook for Families Facing Military Separation,* Colorado Springs, Colorado: David C. Cook, 2005, 286.

Practical suggestions and checklists to help families prepare for deployment.

Hightower, Kathy, and Holly Scherer. *Help, I'm a Military Spouse—I Get a Life Too! How to Craft a Life for You as You Move with the Military.* Washington, DC: Potomac Books Inc., 2007, 198.

Practical suggestions for new military spouses and those contemplating becoming a military spouse.

Lange, Janel. *The Treasure of Staying Connected for Military Couples.* Kingsport, Tennessee: Serviam, 2004, 83.

A waiting wife's advice for maintaining a good relationship despite the stresses of military life, including separation during deployment.

Hines, Sherry. *Homefires: War through the Eyes of a Military Wife.* Fort Campbell, Kentucky: Sherry Hines, 2003, 84.

Another account of a military wife's year while her spouse is deployed.

X References

Waddell, Marshele Carter. *Hope for the Home Front: Winning the Emotional and Spiritual Battles of a Military Wife.* Birmingham, Alabama: New Hope, 2003, 172.

An experienced wife of a navy SEAL shares her faith and methods of coping with her spouse's military service.

Dumler, Elaine Gray. *I'm Already Home...Again—Keeping Your Family Close While on Assignment or Deployment.* Westminster, Colorado: Frankly Speaking, 2006, 106.

Practical suggestions and resources for surviving during deployment.

Booher, Tiffany A. *Spouses Also Serve.* Mustang, Oklahoma: Tate Publishing and Enterprises, 2007, 143.

One woman's account of life as a military wife and how she coped with deployment.

Pace, Brenda, and Carol McGlothlin. *Medals Above My Heart: The Rewards of Being a Military Wife.* Nashville, Tennessee: B&H Publishing Group, 2004, 123.

A little book that combines practical suggestions as well as examples of how two women successfully coped with the stresses of being military wives with the help of their strong Christian faith.

Armstrong, Keith, LCSW, Suzanne Best, PhD, and Paula Domenici, PhD. *Courage After Fire: Coping Strategies for Troops Returning from Iraq and Afghanistan and Their Families.* Berkeley, California: Ulysses Press, 2006, 239.

Practical help for veterans and families making the adjustment to one another and, for the veteran, to civilian life, after deployment.

Dawalt, Sara. *365 Deployment Days: A Wife's Survival Story*. Austin Texas: Bridgeway Books, 2007, 127.

The story of a military wife's year while her husband was deployed. Waiting wives will identify with her feelings and her experience.

Thompson, Jessie. *Behind the Doors of Reality: Tears of a Military Wife: A Mother's Testimonial.* New York, Lincoln, Shanghai: iUniverse Inc., 2006, 92.

Domestic violence leading to the death of her daughter.

Redmond, Jessica. *A Year of Absence: Six Women's Stories of Courage, Hope, and Love.* St. Paul, Minnesota: Elva Resa, 2005, 228.

Six military wives whose husbands are deployed to Iraq. The author's husband was deployed as well.

Carroll, Andrew, ed. *Operation Homecoming: Iraq, Afghanistan, and the Home Front, in the Words of U.S. Troops and Their Families*. New York: Random House, 2006, 386.

A project sponsored by the National Endowment for the Arts. Famous writers visited military bases and helped soldiers tell their stories.

Mock, Janelle H. *Portraits of the Toughest Job in the Army: Voices and Faces of Modern Army Wives.* New York, Lincoln, Shanghai: I Universe Inc., 2007, 234.

The experiences of more than twenty army wives.

Online Resources

Listed below are a few of the many sites available for soldiers, veterans, and their families. You can locate many more online. There are links to specific problems and resources available to help with them.

www.dougbey.com

You can contact me at my website, and I'll do my best to respond.

www.milspouse.com

Information for military spouses, glossary of military terms available here.

http://copingstratagiescd.com

Go to this site for help reducing stress. This is a recording used by army chaplains to help soldiers relax.

www.Cinchouse.com

Where military members and their families are commanders in chief. Information about deployment.

www.nmfa.org

National Military Family Association Inc. Private organization to resolve issues of concern to military families.

www.battlemind.org

Suggestions to help soldiers and families cope with the stresses associated with deployment.

www.militaryonesource.com

Mental health resources for soldiers and families, links with many other helpful sites.

www.al-anon.alateen.org

Support for families, adult children, and friends of alcoholics.

www.alcoholics-anonymous.org

Alcoholics Anonymous, a self-help group for alcoholics.

www.apa.org/pubinfo/anger.html

Information on anger management from the American Psychological Association.

www.childhelpusa.org/programs_hotline.htm

Twenty-four-hour hotline to help locate resources for abused children or children at risk to be abused in your area.

www.seamlesstransition.va.gov

VA website for returning veterans to locate closest VA facilities.

Online Resources

www.va.gov/rcs/index.htm

Counseling centers for veterans and families.

www.deploymentguide.com

Information on deployment for soldiers and families.

www.ncptsd.va.gov

National Center for PTSD, which provides information for soldiers and families on PTSD.

www.gottman.com

Website on relationships and parenting.

www.T.B.I.guide.com

Information for traumatic brain injury survivors and their families.

www.saluteheroes.org/redesign

Website to help military service members who are wounded or disabled and their families.

www.samhsa.gov/vets

Information on prevention, treatment, and recovery support for mental and substance use disorders for veterans and their families.

www.vba.va.gov/vba

Veterans Administration benefits.

www.ingramcontent.com/pod-product-compliance
Lightning Source LLC
Chambersburg PA
CBHW061503180526
45171CB00001B/24